MISDIAGNOSIS

A Practicing Physician's Case Study in

HEALTH CARE REFORM

MISDIAGNOSIS

DR. KIPP A. VAN CAMP

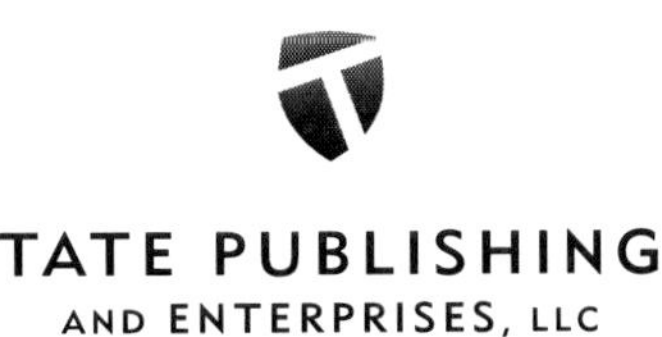

TATE PUBLISHING
AND ENTERPRISES, LLC

Published by Tate Publishing & Enterprises, LLC
127 E. Trade Center Terrace | Mustang, Oklahoma 73064 USA
1.888.361.9473 | www.tatepublishing.com

Tate Publishing is committed to excellence in the publishing industry. The company reflects the philosophy established by the founders, based on Psalm 68:11,
"The Lord gave the word and great was the company of those who published it."

Book design copyright © 2012 by Tate Publishing, LLC. All rights reserved.
Cover & Interior design by Stephanie Mora

Published in the United States of America

ISBN: 978-1-62295-734-7
1. Political Science / Public Policy / Social Services & Welfare
2. Medical / Health Policy
12.08.20

TABLE OF CONTENTS

FOREWORD

SHOULD DOCTORS EVER SPEAK OUT
ON POLITICS AND POLICY?

It's a more controversial question than it may seem at first glance. Dr. Kipp A. Van Camp wants you to read what he has to say, even though he knows he is likely to take some heat from his profession and risks a potential bruising from those who disagree with him.

You'd think that we'd welcome the wisdom and opinions of the very professionals on the frontlines of medicine – those same professionals that we trust with our lives, and the lives of children and parents. But most physicians have been told -whether overtly or through more subtle pressures – to shut up and just get on with the practice of medicine. And when they do speak out, we don't listen.

A survey conducted by the Doctor Patient Medical Association in Summer 2012 revealed that more than 1 out of 3 doctors is hesitant to voice opinions about healthcare politics or policies because of concern about reactions from their hospital administrators, colleagues, and patients. So while we seek out physicians' opinions on medicine, why are so many reluctant to listen to them when it comes to the public policy that drives the medical system?

Much of that disapproval comes from the medical profession itself. Traditionally, physicians have been imbued with the attitude that speaking out is unprofessional, and to be avoided lest one be pegged as a "publicity hound."

The other groups that want doctors to hush up are the politicians and the policymakers. Only a hand-picked few were included in the debate on the massive healthcare reform that eventually brought us the "Patient Protection and Affordable Care Act" of

2010. And when more doctors tried to tell their own American Medical Association that they had problems with the Act, the AMA shut them down, refusing even to allow their own House of Delegates to consider a Resolution opposing the Act.

And when physicians do step up, the results frequently go horribly wrong, resulting in personal attacks and backlash against the messenger. Maybe that's because of the way that physicians are portrayed by a popular media that views them as arrogant, rich, and insensitive. A report produced by the Freedom Forum at Vanderbilt University concluded that "the news media don't trust doctors."

So where did the media come up with this picture of the uncaring physician? One has only to look as far as Washington DC and its environs.

For almost 20 years, I've dragged myself to panel after panel of medical experts at government agencies. I've listened to their testimony. I've read their almost-unreadable reports. They come from an alphabet-soup of agencies, with names like the "National Committee on Vital and Health Statistics" or "Agency for Healthcare Research and Quality." Rarely do the names of these influential agencies include the words "patient" or "doctor."

But what is even more distressing is who makes up these agencies and who their medical experts are. In this world, the "Mud Phuds" rule. These are the M.D.s who also have a Ph.D., usually in the area of "public health" which views the systems as more important than the individual patient. Yes, they are "doctors", but they are usually "physicians" in name-only. Many have never actively practiced medicine or placed their hands on a patient since they were in training. Some also end up with "J.D" after their names, making these doctor-lawyers some of the scariest, overeducated people in the country. They are administrators and number-crunchers, and they are the ones driving healthcare reform and medical policy in this country.

Dr. Kipp A. Van Camp is a Washington insider or agency "expert." Instead, he is a physician in the truest sense of the word.

A real, practicing doctor who has listened to, looked in the eyes of, and put his healing hands on patients for more than twenty-five years. His first responsibility is to his patients – not to the "system."

Dr. Kipp's common-sense analysis of the current state of "reform" initiatives shreds the doubletalk of any of the government toadies and "Mud Phuds." In plain language, he reveals the sometimes "Kafka-esque" nightmare of the current healthcare system largely brought about by government meddling, and explains why more government meddling is almost certainly destined to fail to bring any positive changes.

Our 2012 survey also showed that 83% of doctors think about quitting medicine entirely because of the current changes in the system. Will they all quit? Of course not, but that tells us we have a lot of unhappy doctors. When doctors are unhappy, it's bad for patients. The Doctor Patient Medical Association was founded to bring doctors and patients together to work for solutions. That's exactly what *Misdiagnosis: A Practicing Physician's Case Study in Health Care Reform* does. Dr. Kipp speaks for every physician in this country who sees his profession hanging by a tenuous thread, and fears that we'll soon see freedom of choice for doctors and patients replaced with a centralized and corporatized system where the doctors can do little to fight for their patients.

At the beginning, I asked if doctors should speak out, and when they do, why we don't pay heed. Dr. Kipp is one we should pay attention to, and is a must-read for both physicians and patients. We may not like his prognosis but our lives are at stake - *as well as our freedom.*

—KATHRYN A. SERKES—

Co-Founder, Doctor Patient Medical Association

INTRODUCTION

oes it bother you that it now costs $100 to fill up your vehicle with gas? Are you worried how you will be able to afford to fill up your car? Do you ever wonder how you will make your ends meet? Have you considered giving in and selling your gas-guzzling SUV, even though you love the comfort, safety, and style of your ride? Would you consider a Chevrolet Volt? The president would like for you to consider a Volt. Do you suppose the Secret Service or the federal or state government agents who have SUVs will be trading them in for Volts? Probably not! Why should they? It's not their money they're spending!

If these questions about the vast effects that gasoline and oil prices have on you and your family have crossed your mind, just think how worried you would be if you were sick and unable to afford to get the medical care you needed. It's been said if you have your health, you have everything. The converse has also been suggested: If you don't have your health, you don't have anything. Anyone who has faced illness understands this axiom to be true.

Have you ever been sick? Have you or a loved one ever faced a critical or life-threatening illness? Did it progress to the point where you asked yourself how you would pay for the treatment? One of the universal truths in life is that each of us—if we live long enough—will become a patient. At some time in our lives we will all need medical care.

Two-and-a-half years ago I started a medical show on the radio. During this one-hour a week program interesting topics in medicine are discussed, ranging from specific ailments and diseases, to preventative techniques and therapies, to ethical medical decisions any one of us may face at any given time. Even though these various topics have been well received, one particular subject has repeatedly aroused an exhausted and worn-out public lighting up the switch board: health care reform. Having completed over one-hundred twenty-five different shows, at least thirty times during the past year, numerous experts in medicine and in legislative policy were joined by my listeners in discussing our nation's health care system. And each time we ventured into this discussion, the audience was immediately engaged.

Here's what I observed: Whereas the other shows were entertaining, informative, and enlightening and generated a moderate level of interest, health care reform triggered a frenzy of interest and involvement. Our prepared shows on nationalized health care quickly turned into town hall discussions on the radio. Simply broaching the topic of health care reform, even on a superficial level, triggered intense reactions from my listening audience. The callers' comments and questions revealed genuine concern and even real fear for their own personal health and any treatment they may receive now or in the future. The conclusion was that American's have deep feelings regarding their health. They want security, affordability, and accessibility. They want the benefits of technology. Most scientists recognize that the greatest advances in medicine in the history of the world have happened in the last twenty-five years. The American people want access to the latest and the greatest medical therapies available. And they don't want a third party deciding if, when, what, or where they can receive this treatment.

Through these discussions I realized people's visceral responses were of the same intensity as their reactions to oil and gas prices. I recognized people were greatly concerned about how they would afford health care. And I realized that my twenty-plus years in medicine, including seven years in family medicine and seventeen years in radiology, had afforded me a unique perspective and a greater understanding of the real issues facing us as a nation regarding our health care system and the delivery of medical care.

My first book, *Always Allie,* revealed a doctor's insight into the human-animal bond and how pets positively affect our lives. This experience in completing a quality book provided me invaluable insight and instruction on how to successfully write, edit, produce, and publish. Therefore, for my second book, I decided to jump into the health care debate, feet first. Although this is an entirely different genre, I believe you will find this book informative, educational, and entertaining. This is a light-hearted but direct and poignant look at an extremely complex and serious topic that's about to affect each one of us in ways we could not have imagined!

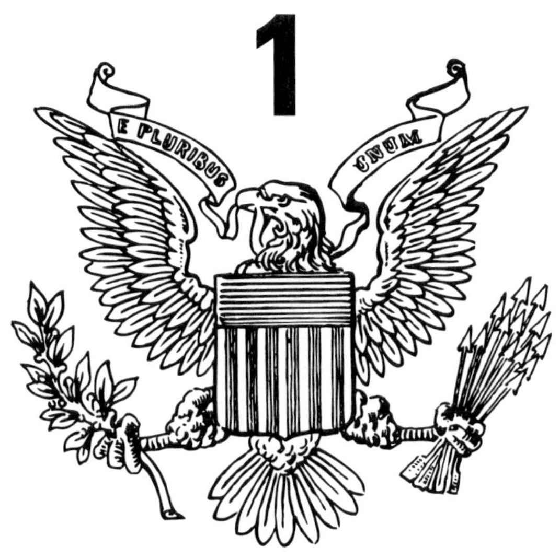

1

BUZZFLASH NEWS ALERT
by House Speaker Nancy Pelosi

Washington, D.C.—Speaker Nancy Pelosi spoke on the House floor tonight in support of historic health insurance reform legislation, (The Patient Protection and Affordable Care Act (PPACA)). The House passed the Senate version of health insurance reform legislation by a vote of 219 to 212. That bill now goes to the president for his signature into law. A second bill, to improve the Senate bill, passed by a vote of 220 to 211 and goes to the Senate. Below are the Speaker's remarks.

"It is with great humility and with great pride that we tonight will make history for our country and progress for the American people. [Applause] Just think—we will be joining those who established Social Security, Medicare, and now tonight health care for all Americans. In doing so, we will honor the vows of our founders, who in the Declaration of Independence said that we are 'endowed by our Creator with certain unalienable rights, that among these are life, liberty and the pursuit of happiness.' This legislation will lead to healthier lives, more liberty to pursue hopes and dreams and happiness for the American people. This is an American proposal that honors the traditions of our country."

Speaking Tuesday to the 2010 Legislative Conference for the National Association of Counties, Pelosi began the windup of her health care pitch by alluding to the controversies over the health care bill and the process by which it has reached its current state: "It's going to be very, very exciting…we [Congress] have to pass the bill so that you can find out what is in it, away from the fog of the controversy."

—By Peter Roff, Posted March 9 2010 [1]

These statements by Nancy Pelosi raise three extremely important issues. First, she stated "we will be joining those who established Social Security, Medicare…" We will take a close look at the histories of Social Security and Medicare. I think you will see that these monstrous social programs strongly go against the free-market system on which our country was founded. I'm not convinced that to be associated with the framers of Medicare and Social Security is such a high honor or compliment. I think you will see my point after reviewing the long-lasting effects of Social Security and specifically Medicare.

Second, in the same speech before Congress, Nancy Pelosi stated that "our founders, who in the Declaration of Independence said that we are 'endowed by our Creator with certain unalienable rights, that among these are life, liberty, and pursuit of happiness.'"[2] Nowhere does it say in the Declaration of Independence that we have a right to health care. I believe this is one of the most important philosophical issues facing our country. And, as a nation, we skipped right over this debate. I'll review some important thoughts on our rights in a moment.

Third, at the 2010 Legislative Conference for the National Association of Counties, Pelosi said "we have to pass the bill so that you can find out what is in it."[3] Many have claimed this was a gaffe, and many believe that gaffes occur only when the truth is inadvertently revealed. This statement speaks loud and clear about what's wrong with Congress and, in turn, what's wrong with America.

Can you imagine in any other walk of life placing your full support behind something about which you had little to no understanding? Would you buy a house based on what the home looks like on the outside or, even worse, having never seen the home at all? Or would you buy a car without test driving it? What if someone removed all the labels from each box and can in a grocery bag and then asked you to buy the groceries? No one in their right mind would do any one of these things. I suppose, in theory, if someone were a great risk taker whose decisions affected only him- or herself, one might say to that person, "Go for it! Good luck to you. If you want to take this risk, that's your business."

But what really makes this disturbing is that every member of Congress has an inherent responsibility to make decisions based on how each individual American will be affected. Yet, Congress passes a bill that Nancy Pelosi has proclaimed as important as Social Security and Medicare, and this health care reform bill will have an influence on the more than 310 million people in this country[4]. And Congress passes this monstrous bill without having read its entirety or having studied its details or the lasting effect it will have on America. This is shameful. In my line of work, that would also be considered negligent.

Maybe Congress should have malpractice insurance. If the bill fails to provide health care benefits to any one of its recipients, should Congress be held liable?

To gain an understanding of our national social programs, we should review the history of Social Security and Medicare. The implementation of both programs was with good intentions. However, as the saying goes, "The road to hell is paved with good intentions"!

HISTORY OF AMERICAN HEALTH CARE

In 1934, President Franklin Delano Roosevelt appointed the Committee on Economic Security (CES). This committee was responsible for creating a system to provide income for the elderly and the disabled. Unlike Ronald Reagan, who believed that we should not look to the government to solve our problems because the government *is* the problem, President Roosevelt believed just the opposite: We should not only look to the government, we should appoint it to solve our problems. In 1935, the CES gave their report to President Roosevelt, recommending a national program that would provide income for the elderly and the disabled. This plan became known as the Social Security Act (SSA). Congress made this a law on August 14, 1935[5].

Specifically, this was a social insurance program that provided a monthly benefit to individuals age sixty-five and older who were no longer working. The monthly benefit was paid to the primary worker when he or she retired, and the amount paid was based on the individual's payroll tax contributions. The SSA also provided unemployment insurance, aid to dependent children, and grants to states for medical care. The Social Security Board was also established and in charge of implementing and overseeing this social program.

Over the years, there have been numerous changes to the system. The program was modified to include benefits to the spouse or minor children of a retired worker. A survivor benefit was added and is paid to the family if a covered coworker dies prematurely. A cost of living adjustment (COLA) was added to the program. The retirement age for men and women was reduced to sixty-two, with a reduced monthly benefit for those choosing to retire early.

Like virtually every one of the government programs, the initial costs to fund the program were underestimated; Social Security was no exception. In 1975, the first official recognition of its failure came from a report by the US Department of the Treasury stating that the amount of money collected from Social Security payroll taxes would not be sufficient to cover the Social Security payments to the recipients, and this shortfall would occur by 1979.[6] The one consistent solution that Congress usually relies on when a program comes up short and needs more money is to increase taxes for working Americans. Not only did Congress raise taxes, they also decreased the monthly benefits to each Social Security recipient and discontinued or froze the COLA at the current rate. Each of these changes was made in an attempt to save Social Security.

In their individual lives, when they realize one of their personal plans or ideas has failed, most rational people admit their failures, learn from their mistakes, and scrap their original plan for a better idea. But that approach is too logical for a government. Instead of scrapping the failed program, Congress, like they do with nearly all their failures, propped up Social Security with more money (confiscated from "Joe Taxpayer"), and they decreased the promised benefits to each individual recipient. What is so audacious about this small group of people running such social programs is that they were the ones who made the decisions for Social Security and yet they pass their failures to those individuals who are paying for the program (and ultimately Congress's failures, too). Where else in life does the person who is paying the bill get stiffed for less money than he or she paid in?

The history of Medicare has some similar themes and commonalities with Social Security. President Roosevelt's CES was originally in charge of following up Social Security with a national health insurance plan. The original report from the CES to President Roosevelt stated that after Social Security was approved, a health insurance plan would be forthcoming. This statement caused such public outcry that President Roosevelt decided to postpone the health insurance issue, fearing that it could jeopardize the future of Social Security. The Social Security Board was originally named the Social Insurance Board; however, this was changed in order to delete all reference to health. Even in 1935, the general public understood just how important it was to keep the government's rationing hands off of health care.[7]

Even with the strong opposition, the politicians were not deterred. After all, don't let a definitive outcry from Joe Taxpayer hinder your willingness and determination to shape a once free-market system into a massive social state. With a sleight of hand, President Roosevelt appointed an Interdepartmental Committee to Coordinate Health and Welfare Activities (ICCHWA) within less than a year. This committee established a subcommittee (the Technical Committee) on medical care whose members decided in a private conference that "it would be desirable to formulate a comprehensive National Health Program."[8] Thus began a social health program that would culminate in a national health care system nearly eighty years later.

The Technical Committee published its report in February 1938 recommending a "general program of medical care, paid for either through general taxation or social insurance contributions as well as federal support for hospital expansion, disability insurance, public health services—including maternal and child health—and state programs for the 'medically needy.'" With this groundwork properly laid, health care legislation was introduced in virtually every session of Congress from 1939 onward. The American Medical Association (AMA) strongly opposed national health insurance, claiming it was socialized medicine.[9] They received overwhelming public support. In predictable governmental fashion, Congress and President Roosevelt would not be persuaded, and they persisted year after year with health care legislation.

Even a 1942 *Fortune* poll indicated strong public opposition, with 76.3 percent of the public stating that the government should not provide free medical care.[10] Once again, the elitists in Congress knew what was better for the general public than did the actual people themselves. In 1944, the Social Security Board specifically recommended to Congress that compulsory national health insurance be made part of the Social Security system.

The national health care advocates carried out an extensive media campaign in an attempt to convince the public. In 1942, *Fortune* magazine ran an important article that was decidedly in favor of the proposed health program. When Harry Truman became president in 1945, he submitted the first-ever presidential message devoted exclusively to health care.[11]

In 1950-51, a key development occurred in Congress: The Democrats suffered net losses in the House and Senate. Key congressional leaders in the Social Security Administration who had been proponents of national health insurance from the beginning came to believe that universal health insurance could not be passed. So, they lowered their sights to focus on a program for just the elderly and the disabled—and just like that, the notion of Medicare was born.[12] They never totally forgot about a universal program but came to believe that a smaller, more specific version of the same idea would suffice, for the time being.

National health insurance proponents continued to receive strong opposition from the AMA and the medical community; however, they remained persistent. With the continued drumbeat of societal opinion against such a program, they decided upon an incremental approach. If they could simply break the program into pieces and pass the legislation one small part at a time, they could ultimately succeed. And succeed they did, first with a disability program added to Social Security in 1956.[13] In 1957, with disability coverage in place, the American Federation of Labor and Congress of Industrial Organizations (AFL-CIO) jumped into the discussion, recommending compulsory health insurance for its union brethren. Again, the strategy of incrementalism was used, adding a small piece of health care legislation to an already existing program, incrementally, one part at a time. The AFL-CIO formulated a bill proposing hospital, surgical, and nursing home benefits for Social Security recipients. The bill went before Congress and was barely defeated.

Sensing they were close to succeeding, proponents brought the next bill before Congress in 1960. The Kerr-Mills Bill[14] proposed a needs-based program of medical assistance for the aged poor. Congress hoped this would be a limited way to deal with this issue of health insurance, and so the opposition party agreed, assuming passage would finally end this two-plus-decade debate. The bill passed by a slim margin.

As we have seen so many times with the Democrat Party over the years, giving in and allowing them a lesser version of their ideal program, whatever it happens to be, doesn't usually bring the issue to an end. Instead, passage of the limited version of their social legislation only fuels their drive to press on with a larger, more aggressive plan. After passage of the limited Kerr-Mills Bill, this proved true. In 1961 and again in 1963, the King-Anderson Bill went before Congress, proposing compulsory health care insurance for the aged.[15] Even with President John F. Kennedy's support, the King-Anderson Bill was defeated by slim margins.

BIRTH OF MEDICARE

Instead of being discouraged and letting the universal health insurance program die a natural death, the Democrats were renewed and invigorated. After a resounding Democrat victory in the November 1964 general elections, the bill that became known as Medicare was passed by Congress in 1965. It was later believed that Medicare passed because of the incremental passage of one small piece of health care legislation at a time. The bill would provide compulsory hospital insurance financed through the Social Security payroll tax, payable to people over sixty-five years of age. After a small hospital deductible, hospital bills would be covered for sixty days. Ancillary coverage was to be provided for sixty days of nursing home care. Physicians' services outside the hospital, catastrophic illness that lasted more than sixty days, and therapeutic drugs were not covered.

After the dust had settled and the bill had been enacted, it became clear that the program was wrought with limitations. In fact, Senator Russell Long (D-LA) asked, Health, Education and Welfare (HEW) Secretary Anthony Celebrezze, who had been instrumental in writing the Medicare bill, "Why do you leave out the real catastrophes, the catastrophic illness?" Celebrezze responded, [16]"The bill was not intended for those that are going to stay in institutions year-in and year-out." Senator Long then replied, "Well, in arguing for your plan you say let's not strip poor old grandma of the last dress she has and of her home and what little resources she has and you bring us a plan that does exactly that unless she gets well in sixty days."

Apparently, whenever the legislature wanted to convince public opinion of Medicare, they used cases like this where a senior had a prolonged illness and was unable to afford the extensive health care needed over a lengthy period. Yet, when the bill was written and ultimately passed, the same scenario they used to gain support was excluded from the bill, another example of the less-than-forthright methods of our corrupt legislature.

As you can see, Medicare was a long time coming. However, like every other social program, regardless of its expense, once it was passed its inefficiencies and failures were here to stay. Why are these monstrosities allowed to become even more bloated and less effective? Why don't we reevaluate these programs, scrap them if they're failing and before they've had thirty or forty years of failures, and then try something else? Why don't we learn from our mistakes and come up with better systems that are more efficient and effective? No, that sounds too logical. Instead, our Congress tweaks, regulates, and adds to the already bloated and ineffective bureaucracies, cramming their failures and their expenses down our throats.

Of course, the proposed bill was insufficient in the legislature's eyes, so over the next forty years Congress added to, rearranged, and revised Medicare. They were perpetually short on money and on their projected budgets, and so America paid for these additions and "miscalculations" in the form of tax increases. The massive social program limped into the twenty-first century. Near the end of the first decade of 2000, it became clear that this time Medicare faced serious shortcomings. For the first time since 1965, Medicare was on the ropes. In 2008, Medicare received income (or collections) of $221 billion but paid out a total of $230 billion in benefits and administrative expenses. This resulted in a deficit of $8 billion for the year. At the end of 2008, the "trust fund" held $318 billion. Following this trend, Medicare will be insolvent, including the depletion of the entire trust fund reserves, by the year 2019. So, after chronic mismanagement, Medicare will officially be broke in 2019.[17]

We learn from history. It tends to repeat itself; therefore, if we are paying attention, we can see the signs that signaled our mistakes, and we can prevent the same failures from happening a second time. Yet, even after we realized that Social Security was going broke, we skipped on down the primrose, massive social program path and implemented Medicare without any hint of learning from our mistakes.

How many times must we repeat the same pattern before we realize that a large social program is incapable of providing all the needs (not to mention the many wants) of its recipients? In America, Congress is more than happy to go back to the taxpayer well again and again. And so, whenever a poorly managed social program is underfunded, the taxpayers bail it out. Whenever any social program comes up short on money, Congress resorts to one of only a couple solutions: Increase the amount of money coming in by increasing the taxes of the workers (there's no need to tax the nonworkers; they don't have anything to tax) or decrease the services being provided. In the case of Social Security, Congress decreased the monthly payment, regardless of how much or how long each individual recipient has been contributing. In the case of Medicare, Congress decreased available services but never called this rationing; instead, they claimed these services were uncovered services, even though "uncovered service" is code for "rationed care."

So, when Nancy Pelosi says she's proud to lump the Patient Protection and Affordable Care Act (PPACA) in with the likes of Medicare and Social Security, she's experiencing misplaced hubris. In reality, the public would feel much better about this new health care program if it had no resemblance and no association with Social Security or Medicare.[18]

RIGHT OR PRIVILEGE?

The Declaration of Independence says we are endowed by our Creator with certain unalienable rights … rights afforded the citizens of the United States, not the noncitizens (i.e., aliens). Among these are life, liberty, and the pursuit of happiness.[19] Again, nowhere in this document does it say life, liberty, pursuit of happiness, and *health care*. Let's take a close look at rights vs. privileges.

As a nation, we skipped past the important dialogue on the difference between rights and privileges. There are very few true rights in this life. Our wise founders wanted a country that was unique regarding rights and freedoms. So, when they formed the rights of the citizens of the United States, they said that anyone fortunate enough to be a citizen of the United States had three rights: life, liberty, and pursuit of happiness. Anything else is not a right but a privilege. It may even be a want, but it is not a right.

Let's look even deeper. Every human being who walks the face of this earth has three basics needs or necessities: food, shelter, and clothing. If we expanded this list to include the top five necessities, in the order of importance, one could add education and then health care.

Before I discuss these needs in detail, let's take a moment to review free market vs. Socialism. The free-market system is the most effective and most fair system throughout all of history. No other socioeconomic system has proved as prosperous or as successful. With Socialism, the overall theme is to provide for the well-being of all its citizens. On the surface, this sounds nice. But the problem is that the working class provides all the resources for the nonworking class. As a society, we feel a moral obligation to not allow a person to starve or to lay destitute in the street. The problem isn't the willingness as a society to reach out and provide some assistance to this indigent or needy person; the problem always is how much to provide. Pure Socialism never has a limit. How far should we set our limit? What is the end point? Let me explain.

Free market says people who work should get paid. The amount of their pay should be proportionate to the quality of the service they provide. The availability of the service is also a limiting factor. The price is determined based on how much it would cost to get the same service completed for the same or similar quality.

For example, say I want to build a fence around my yard. Using the free-market approach, I would look to the fence companies to see what it would cost me to build my fence. I would evaluate the quality of the fence companies' work by reviewing other fences they have built. Then, I would make my own decision based on how much money I could commit to the fence project. If I had less money to put into this fence, I could either change the fence to a smaller one or use lesser-quality materials. I could also hire the company who does less-quality work for a lower price. However, if I were seeking a fence in a socialistic system, all fence material, quality of laborers, and time to complete the fence would be the same. I would not be allowed to decide what I could and what I couldn't afford. Instead, the fence companies would be managed by a central governing fence company and see to it that all fences were similar and the same cost to build.

For another example, let's look at the minimum wage. In a free-market system, the wage is determined based on the number of workers, the employer's ability to pay them, and the quality of their work. The workers are paid a price based on supply and demand. In a socialized state, the workers are guaranteed a minimum wage assigned by the governing body, which in our country is Congress. Again, on the surface, this sounds good. Why shouldn't workers be paid at least a certain amount (i.e., minimum wage) for their efforts? If a minimum wage is set at $10 an hour, why shouldn't the workers be given a minimum of $12.50 an hour instead? And if $12.50 an hour is given, why shouldn't it be raised to $15, $20, or even $50 an hour? What's the end point? When does it seem fair and appropriate to say, "Well, that minimum is enough"? Should there be a maximum wage, too?

Using this same logic regarding food, shelter, and clothing, how much is enough? How much food is fair and acceptable to provide minimum food consumption? Should the central governing body (Congress) see to it that all citizens are provided three square meals a day? What about snacks? And what about the type and quality of the food? Shouldn't Joe Taxpayer eat steak and potatoes? Why not surf and turf (lobster and steak)? What about caviar? Shouldn't all citizens be given quality food? Who decides what the end point is? Is there a fair and reasonable limit?

What about shelter? Should each citizen be provided a simple room and a roof over their head, or should each be guaranteed the American Dream: a home? How big should the home be? How about three bedrooms, one bathroom, and a two-car garage? Is 1,500 square feet big enough? Why not 2,000 or even 5,000 square feet? What about a swimming pool?

And while we're at it, what about clothing? Should all citizens be guaranteed a shirt, shoes, and pants? Perhaps all should be guaranteed a uniform? Is clothing one of the three basic needs? Is it fair to limit people's clothing? Why shouldn't each person who's a citizen of the United States be provided with brand-name, quality clothing like Pierre Cardin or Gucci?

Can we agree that the fourth basic need is education? We as a nation have already striven to provide an education to all our citizens. Everybody is required to complete the public education provided up to age sixteen. If an individual wishes, he or she will be provided a K–12 education. Why do we stop there? Why shouldn't we provide a college education or at least a vocational education, too? What about quality? I don't even want to get into the shortcomings of the public school system. But, accepting there may be some limitations, why shouldn't each student receive a private K–12 education? And why shouldn't all citizens be guaranteed an Ivy League college education? Why should we limit the amount or quality of the education to the public school system?

The fifth basic need could be health care. If it is, then following this same line of thinking, should all people receive their health care from the Mayo Clinic or the Cleveland Clinic? Why not? Should all citizens receive unlimited health care? Shouldn't this unlimited care include plastic surgery or cosmetic health care, too? Who decides who gets what services and who doesn't?

You can see all the practical— not to mention ethical—dilemmas this philosophy causes. That's why the only real solution lies with the free-market system. When the overseers get out of the way, the consumers are extremely successful at finding the best products and best care for the best price.

Perhaps (and this is a big perhaps) there is a basic level of each of these five basic needs that we might be willing to provide each citizen. But once you begin this type of solution, you are heading down a slippery slope every time because no one is willing to stick to the basic level. "If this basic need is good, then just a little bit more is better," is the argument that's always raised. And once you add to the most basic level of service only one time, you will always modify it again.

Maybe we could guarantee each person three square meals a day. Oh, that's right, we already do that with food stamps. Well, then, maybe we could guarantee all citizens a roof over their head and shelter from storms. Oh, that's right, we already do that, too, with government housing. Just how are these two programs doing?

The problem is that we skipped the most important discussion of all: We went past the "what are privileges" discussion and right to the "what are rights" discussion. Once you declare it is your right to have food, shelter, clothing, education, and health care, you head straight down the "class envy" path. It is inevitable. Why does he get that food while I'm stuck with this? How come he lives in that house and I have this? You see, once you head down this path of labeling each of these needs as rights, you completely remove personal responsibility and free market and create a dependent welfare state.

We, as a society and a political system, need to have this discussion on what constitutes privileges vs. rights and a basic level of assistance that is fair and reasonable. What is the realistic minimum? (Again, this entire line of thinking is flawed.) Until we engage in these tough discussions, and until we can come to some reasonable conclusions, we will continue to fail miserably. We will run up huge deficits, placing the cost burden on the working class, expecting the workers to provide for their needs as well as those of their nonworking fellow citizens. We will continue to be bogged down with regulations and bureaucracies, never really improving any of our citizens' quality of life or their human conditions.

Now, let's briefly discuss the statement "we have to pass the bill so that you can find out what is in it." There's so much wrong and not much right with this statement. Why are the bills so vast and extensive? The PPACA is greater than 2,400 pages long, and that doesn't even include the thousands of pages of regulations currently being written by US Health and Human Services (HHS) Secretary Kathleen Sebelius.[20] Why are these bills so complex? The PPACA is just like our tax code, which is so bloated and complicated that no two certified public accountants can prepare a complex tax return and come up with the same figures at the completion. If and when there's a simpler, fairer, more logical solution, Congress always selects the more complicated one. Do you ever ask yourself why? It appears the answer to this question lies in illusions.

The more complex and extensive any legislation is, the easier it is to confuse, deny, regulate, and hide details within the pages of the vast minutiae. Why not follow the adage "Keep it simple, stupid (KISS)"?

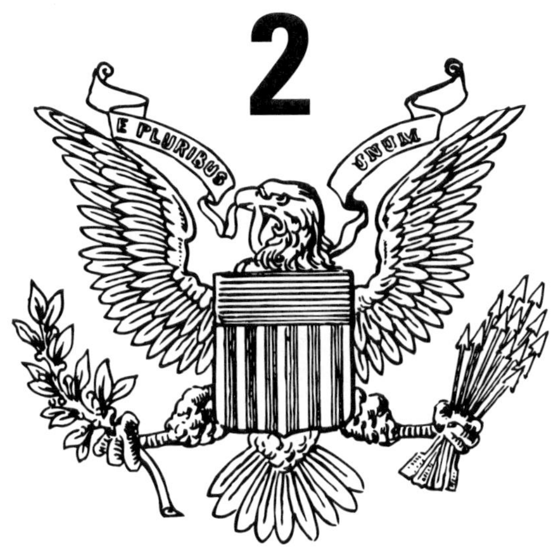

2

WILL CONGRESS EVER GET A HANDLE ON CONTROLLING SPENDING?

et's take a moment to look at some of the specific statistics regarding Medicare, Medicaid, Social Security, and health insurance. Each of the following numbers and percentages come from the Congressional Budget Office (CBO). Currently, 85 percent of Americans have health insurance. There are about 310 million Americans. The breakdown of who is on what type of insurance is as follows: Of the 85 percent, 60 percent receive their insurance from their employer. Another 9 percent are either self-employed, unemployed with some wealth, or retired but too young to qualify for Medicare and so they buy their insurance directly from the insurance companies.[1] The remaining 31 percent are currently on Medicare or Medicaid. Multiple sources state that there are 34 million American citizens without health insurance.[2] If you simply take our population of 310 million citizens and accept that 85 percent of them have health insurance, then you would calculate that the 15 percent of this country without insurance would equal about 46 million people.[3] Also, there are 27 million employers in America.[4]

The president has the audacity to tell us that under the PPACA there will be a decrease in health care expenses. He also says that we will pay for much of the plan by cutting out the fraud and abuse within the Medicare system.[5] But on top of all this talk on decreasing costs and Medicare expenses, his most far-fetched declaration is that we will also cut the national debt by $138 billion over the next decade. In 1966, the cost of Medicare was close to $3 billion; in 2009, it was $427 billion (not including the one-time injection of $255 billion from the Stimulus Bill). The chief actuary for the centers for Medicare and Medicaid (CMS) reports that the cost will reach $311 billion over the next ten years, not decrease or stay the same. The CBO reports that Medicare will be underfunded by $36.6 trillion over the next seventy-five years. That's almost $500 billion per year, which is more than double what the chief actuary for Medicare and Medicaid suggests.[6] The president claims the deficit will be reduced by $138 billion over the next ten years, but the CBO says the truth is that there will be an increase in the federal budget deficit by $230 billion over the next decade from 2012 to 2021.[7] The House Budget Committee paints an even more dismal picture, saying the federal deficit will increase by $701 billion over the first ten years from 2010 to 2020.[8] Douglas Holtz-Eakin, PhD, president of the American Action Forum and former director of the CBO, says that the health care reform legislation will raise the federal debt by $562 billion over the next decade.[9] So, whom are you going to trust? Which numbers are you going to believe?

Here is the truth, and it's something you are not hearing from our government officials, government agencies, or our media: Modern-day American government officials do NOT decrease expenditures. They do NOT cut budgetary spending. They are incapable of spending less. Whenever our government gets their hands on any of our money, they spend it. If they can't confiscate enough money in the form of taxes, then they print new money. For the hard-working Americans who struggle daily to make ends meet and try to get ahead, it is insulting and infuriating that their government leaders have spent them into oblivion.

A FISCAL CONSCIENCE

Decades ago, the government had a small modicum of integrity. They truly respected the taxpayer, attempted to be cognizant of the money we sent to Washington in the form of our taxes, and tried to be responsible with spending. Those days are long gone. The last time we even approached a balanced budget in which the government used our tax dollars effectively and where each program was paid for and our big social programs were appropriately funded was back in the 1950s. The old saying "familiarity breeds contempt" must be true, as the elected governmental officials over the past sixty years became complacent and careless with our money. When a small group of elected officials (435 members of the US House of Representatives; 100 US senators; a president; a vice president; and, if you want to be generous, 50 governors for a total of 587 people at any one time)[10] are able to spend my money and your money in whatever fashion they see fit, it stands to reason that they will screw it up. It's really easy to spend someone else's money! And the safety net of the printing press doesn't help the situation!

If I had been an elected official anytime in the past sixty years in America, I would currently be absolutely ashamed of the misuse and overextension of the American people's money. Everywhere you turn, another government agency is bankrupt, another state is in financial ruin, and another key program is asking for more money. This is at all levels of government, from city to state to federal. In many ways, these actions should be looked at as treasonous. The entire government in the country with the greatest wealth in the history of the world is flat broke. How can that even be possible, except for overspending, fraud, abuse, corruption, arrogance, and ignorance? Oh, sure, the freethinkers will say that's why we have elections, to vote out the bad officials. Anyone who has been responsible for creating this massive and incomprehensible debt should be held accountable. Frankly, it's become so bad that kicking these officials out or not re-electing them isn't good enough. With Enron, we sent the corrupt to prison; with any other bankrupt company, we close them down with significant repercussions. Therefore, why not line up all these 587 people (at any one time) and place them in stockades outside our statehouses and our Congress? Perhaps we could even hang signs around their necks that identify them as thieves, crooks, or at least fools.

Instead, we reward them (or at least allow them to reward themselves) with better pension plans than the rest of us and higher levels of and greater access to the best health care in the world at a cheaper price. We reward them with an equal or greater-than cost-of-living raise every year, something most of us haven't seen in quite a while. In fact, doctors have been experiencing Medicare cuts and decreasing payment from insurance for years. We American citizens treat these irresponsible politicians like they are nobility. We cheer when they approach. We block off the roads for their motorcades to pass. We grant them access to airplanes and the greatest modes of transportation. These folks are placed on a pedestal as if they were the brightest and wisest of society. And yet, the so-called brightest have bankrupted us at all levels of government.

The PPACA will lead to the largest expansion of government ever in the United States. I think I've laid out some rather compelling arguments why we don't want the government to get any larger or allow them to have any more control over any other areas of our lives. Congress can't manage the PPACA efficiently. Remember, it is more than 2,409 pages long, and the Senate version included another 153 additional pages for a total Senate version of 2562 pages.

If I asked you which is the most complex government agency or what has the most complicated rules and regulations in our current government, what comes to mind? I would suspect that many people would say it's the US tax code or the Internal Revenue Service (IRS). If I asked a number of people what governmental agency has the most power in America, other than the FBI or the CIA, I suspect many would again say it's the IRS. So, the agency that has unbelievable power is placed in charge of one of the most complicated pieces of legislation ever passed, Title 26, the US tax code. This ridiculously complex piece of legislation has 3,458 pages and 5.6 million words,[11] seven times as many as the Bible.

And now, following suit, the brightest people in our society have created another bloated piece of legislation that is so complicated that they have to pass it so that they can see what's in it. It has 2,400 pages of laws, mandates, and requirements. But that's only the beginning. There are the thousands of pages of regulations that are being developed by our HHS department. The woman in charge of this department and these regulations and who has equal or greater power regarding your health is Kathleen Sebelius, who isn't an elected official. She was appointed by the president and is accountable only to him.[12] She's not even in health care. She was the insurance commissioner of Kansas and then became that state's governor. Why on earth should she have such power over our health care system? Wouldn't you want someone in there who understands the current health system, who recognizes our many strengths, and who identifies our numerous shortcomings? An absolute requirement for the HHS secretary should be a health care background and so many years working in the trenches actually administering patient care.

Don't believe it when you hear the news out of Washington, from or our media, or from the president himself that says this will be affordable or that this will actually cost us less than the current system. It will be extremely expensive. That's what our government does: They spend our money. They overpromise and overbudget.

They create levels and levels of bureaucracy. A December 11, 2009 *USA Today* article showed the average salaries for jobs in the public sector vs. private sector. The average federal worker makes $71,206 a year, whereas the average private sector worker makes $40,331 a year.[13] That's over $30,000 more per government employee each year when compared with the private sector worker.

Simply following this logic, the president has stated that there will be 16,000 more IRS agents to uncover, discover, and prosecute health care providers, insurance companies, and pharmaceutical and device companies for fraud and abuse of Medicare. If these workers make the average public sector salary of $71,206, that's about $1.1 billion.[14] Also, the goal is to educate and place 16,000 new primary care physicians (PCPs)[15] into practice. According to the American Academy of Family Physicians (AAFP) and according to Simply Hired, the average salary for a family physician (FP) in 2011 is $113,000.[16] This is $1.8 billion in additional expenses. There are over 159 new regulatory committees that are being appointed and selected as we speak. These new committees are said to account for at least 1,700 new jobs.[17] When the president speaks of how the PPACA is creating new jobs, these are all public sector jobs, and all are all ultimately at the expense of the American taxpayer.

No, the PPACA will not make health care more affordable. It will not make the health system more efficient. It certainly will not cut the deficit. New government programs never do!

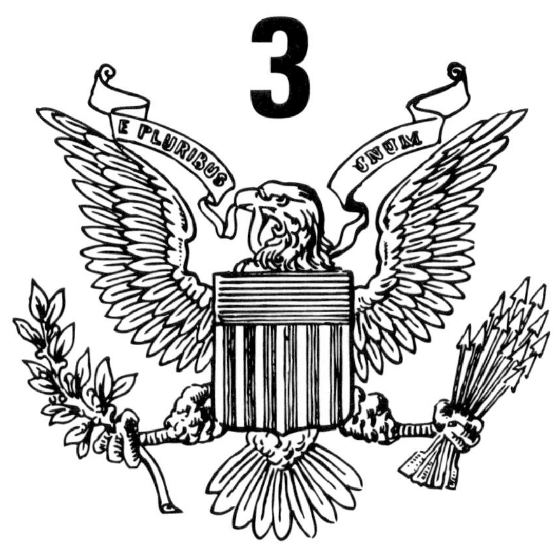

3

WHAT'S NOT IN THE PPACA?

It's time to begin dissecting the bill to see what it includes. What are the details? The idiom "the devil is in the details" may actually be true. But before we look at all the regulations and requirements, there's one more discussion to be had. It's the greatest omission with the most potential gain regarding controlling costs in the PPACA.

Suppose you awaken with a bellyache. You toughen it out for the first part of the day; however, as the day progresses, you continue to feel pretty lousy. Your stomach hurts to the touch. Because you are nauseated, you don't eat anything all day. Around six o'clock in the evening you give in and decide to head to the emergency department at your local hospital. After filling out the many pieces of paper, and after being in the waiting room for twenty minutes, you are finally escorted back to the patient area and placed in an emergency examination bed. The nurse comes in and begins to ask you questions. After several minutes of questions and exam forms, she takes your vital signs, writes something on your chart, and then leaves. Before you can see the doctor, the phlebotomist—the person who draws your blood—comes in. He takes a couple of vials of your blood and then leaves a cup behind and asks you to give him a urine specimen. During your intake questioning, the nurse asks, "Have you had any chest pain?" You answer, "Sure, maybe a little." Since your belly began hurting, you have had a minimal amount of discomfort in your lower chest. Before you know it, a technician arrives and hooks you up to an electrocardiograph machine, which produces an electrocardiogram (ECG) that shows your heart rhythm. Before the ECG is completed, another technician shows up to take x-ray pictures. She takes a picture of your chest and two pictures of your abdomen, known as an acute abdominal series.

The nurse reappears and says the doctor will be in momentarily. Fifteen minutes later, the doctor comes in for the first time. She talks with you about your symptoms for about five minutes and then proceeds to examine you. She listens to your heart and your stomach. She looks in your ears, eyes, and mouth. She palpates over your neck and your belly. Upon completion, she asks, "Have you had a bowel movement today?" You're embarrassed by this but answer, "No." She presses further and asks, "Did you have one yesterday?" You respond with "I don't think so." She asks, "Is that normal for you?" You say, "No, it isn't. I'm pretty darn regular." She announces, "We'll have to do a rectal exam." Before you realize what's going on, a gloved finger is forced into your rectum. The K-Y jelly is cold and wet. "Everything's fine there," the doctor reassures you.

As she's about to leave your exam room, she turns and says, "I'll bet you're just constipated, but we shall soon find out." She leaves. You sit there feeling awkward and somehow violated by these personal and probing questions. About forty-five minutes later, the nurse returns. "We need to take you over to radiology for a CT scan," she tells you. She gives you a nasty-tasting bottle of white liquid to drink. You begin sipping it down while she pushes you in your gurney out of the emergency department and down the hall to the radiology department.

After you polish off the bottle of liquid, the computed tomography (CT) technician says, "I'll have to wait one hour before I can take your CT scan." You ask, "Does it usually take this long?" She replies, "Usually they make people wait for two hours after drinking the white contrast, but the doctor in the ER is more lenient than most, so you're lucky." You aren't feeling that lucky right now.

Precisely one hour later, the CT tech reappears and wheels you into the CT room. "Please slide onto the CT table," she requests. She starts an IV and hooks it to a machine. "Lie very still," she says, "and follow the instructions given by the computer." A few seconds after she leaves the room, a computerized voice says, "Take in a deep breath, now blow it out, take in a deep breath, and hold your breath." The machine begins to make a whirring sound. As the table begins to move you through the x-ray tube, you feel coldness going up your arm and into your shoulder as the automatic injector machine connected to your IV injects IV contrast into your vein. It's a strange sensation that passes as quickly as it occurs. The table stops, and you are completely inside the x-ray tube. You are not panicked, as the tube is wide open on both ends. The table moves in and out a couple more times then comes to a stop in the original starting position. The CT tech enters the room again and says, "We're finished. Please slide over to the gurney." You accommodate her without any discussion. She disconnects you from the machine but leaves the IV in your vein in case you need medicine in the emergency department. "What did you see?" you ask her. She says, "I'm the tech. The radiologist needs to make the interpretation. We should have that in twenty to thirty minutes."

You wait in your emergency department room for another forty-five minutes until the doctor appears. "Like I suspected," she reports, "I think you're constipated. All your tests are normal. Your labs are fine. Your urinalysis was clear. And your x-rays and your

CT scan were read as normal. So, you don't have appendicitis." You ask, "Why did we do all these tests if you thought it was appendicitis?" She says, "Well, we had to be sure. I didn't want to miss a hot appendix or anything else bad." She then discharges you to home with instructions to take some milk of magnesia. You do, and by the next day you are back to your normal routine and the bellyache is gone. The doctor was right.

Within a month the bills start to roll in. There's a lab bill and a couple of different hospital bills, including the emergency department charges, the lab charges, and the x-ray charges. Within a couple of days a bill comes from the emergency department doctor. Within two weeks a bill comes from the radiologist. In total, your trip to the emergency department cost your insurance and you a total of $19,500. You are shocked at the cost, especially because your doctor said before many of the tests were performed that you were probably just constipated, and she was indeed correct. What an expensive trip to the hospital to find out you simply needed a laxative.

DEFENSIVE MEDICINE

Does this sound far-fetched or embellished? It's not at all. In fact, it's so accurate it's sobering. Why did the doctor order all these tests? Why didn't she follow her convictions and simply trust her skills? The answer is she was practicing defensive medicine. This is what all of us doctors do. We do it to protect ourselves from being sued. We do it for the patient, too. But we don't have the luxury of doing the most cost-effective action, because for every 1,000 or so cases just like the one above, one of them could actually present with appendicitis, and we risk harming the patient and being sued for missing a diagnosis.

If you're the patient, you don't want your doctor to miss a diagnosis any more than your doctor wants to miss one. But you also don't want to pay for all these unnecessary tests.

POLLING DATA

A University of Connecticut study, believed to be the very first of its kind, polled 900 doctors from Massachusetts and asked them about their use of seven different tests and procedures: plain film x-rays, CT scans, magnetic resonance imaging (MRI) scans, laboratory tests, sonograms, specialty referrals and consultations, and hospital admissions.[1] A total of 83 percent reported practicing defensive medicine, with an average of 18 to 28 percent of tests, referrals, consults, or hospital admissions ordered for defensive reasons. The study estimated that $1.4 billion per year of additional and unnecessary tests were performed in Massachusetts alone. The study results are telling; however, I think the study was inherently flawed. I don't know of a doctor who doesn't practice defensive medicine—the study should have shown that 100 percent of doctors practice it. I suspect some of the doctors were afraid to be completely forthright and honest, as they may have wondered if there were some way of tracking which doctor answered which way and that this could ultimately have a detrimental effect on their practice.

A December 2009 Gallup poll showed that 73 percent of physicians surveyed nationwide said they practiced some form of defensive medicine in the past twelve months to protect themselves from frivolous lawsuits.[2] Jackson Healthcare estimates that $650 billion of the $2.5 trillion spent on health care in 2010 year was spent on unnecessary tests because physicians practiced defensive medicine. This could have the greatest impact of all on decreasing the bloated costs of health care.

We have yet to talk about the other health professionals such as physicians' assistants (PAs) and nurse practitioners (NPs), who we know ob rder significantly more tests and ancillary services than do doctors because of the nature of thcir role in health care delivery.

TORT REFORM

After his state enacted tort reform measures in late 2010, Texas Governor Rick Perry noted that the number of doctors applying to practice medicine in Texas skyrocketed by 57 percent and that tort reforms brought critical specialties to underserved areas. He said that these reforms are real tort reforms that actually improve access to health care.[3] Another research study suggests about $200 billion per year could be saved with legal reform.[4]

After Governor Perry successfully passed tort reform, the state of Texas has seen an increase in the number of physicians practicing in his state. The state government has provided doctors a more conducive system to practice cost effective medicine. At the peril of the other state's this has resulted in a large migration of primary care physicians, obstetricians and neurosurgeons to the state of Texas.

But tort reform is not even included in the PPACA. The president, the Democratic Congress, and the media tell us all the time that this is about patient care and doing the right thing for the patient in the most efficient manner. Yet, when they have a chance to include the one thing that would have the greatest impact on health reform, they refuse to include it in the bill. Why? Why are they dishonest when it comes to genuine reform?

The following was recently published in the *Washington Examiner*: Howard Dean proved last week at Rep. Jim Moran's health care town hall meeting that even a veteran Washington politician can level with people once in a while. The former Vermont governor and Democratic presidential aspirant was a practicing physician before he got into politics, so perhaps we should not be surprised by his explanation for why medical malpractice caps [i.e., tort reform] is not in Obamacare: "The reason tort reform is not in the bill is because the people who wrote it did not want to take on the trial lawyers in addition to everybody else they were taking on. And that's the plain and simple truth."[5] Put otherwise, trial lawyers have effectively bought themselves veto power.

According to OpenSecrets.org, the American Association for Justice (AAJ)—formerly the Association of Trial Lawyers of America—ranks sixth on the list of the top 100 special-interest groups regarding campaign contributions during the past twenty years. The AAJ is the trial lawyers' Washington lobbying group, and 90 percent of its $30.7 million in contributions since 1989 have gone to the Democrats. At the other end of this pay-to-play process in the nation's capital, the AAJ has spent nearly $14 million lobbying Congress since the Democrats won control of both chambers, including $2.3 million thus far in 2011.[6].

The Democratic focus on the plaintiff's bar is even more obvious from campaign contributions listed in *National Journal*'s top fifteen class-action trial attorney firms. David Freddoso and Kevin Mooney of the *Washington Examiner* reported that those firms in 2009 contributed more than $636,000, 99 percent of which went to the Democrats. Employees of those firms have given more than $236,000 to the Democratic Senatorial Campaign Committee in 2011.[7]

Governors such as Rick Perry of Texas and Haley Barbour of Mississippi have enacted tort reform in their states with much success.[8] Capping medical malpractice suits has saved billions of dollars by lowering the cost of insurance for providers and increasing access to quality care for patients.[9] Unless we place a cap on medical malpractice, trial lawyers will make millions of dollars in fees through questionable malpractice cases. You can see why the Democrats absolutely insist that tort reform will NEVER be included in a health reform bill as long as they are in power. Too much of the trial lawyers' monetary donations ends up going to the Democratic president, the DNC, and the Democratic congressional coffers.

As long as the trial lawyers continue to make significant money on questionable cases, and as long as they continue to overwhelmingly support the Democratic Party, we will never see real and lasting health care reform. If these members of Congress were truly genuine about improving the health care system, they would take tort reform head-on. But they aren't interested in real health care reform; it's all talk. Their agenda is to gain more control over the American people and create a single-payer system where we all get our health insurance from a single source: the American government. That is Socialism! And if you don't believe me, you should believe Barney Frank when he said if anyone is discouraged about the possibility of the PPACA not insuring broad enough health care reform, don't be, this is only the of the door to complete reform.

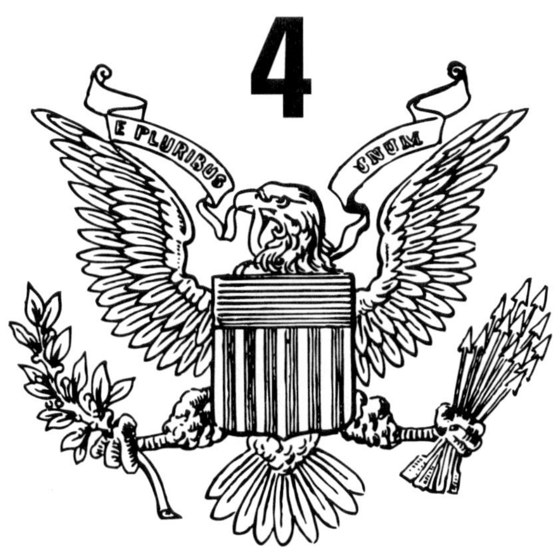

WHAT ABOUT ALL THE UNINSURED?

Apparently, anywhere from 34 million to 50 million Americans do not have health insurance. These people either make too much money to qualify for Medicaid; have taken a risk by believing they are healthy and therefore have elected not to purchase insurance; or have retired early, paid significantly for a Consolidated Omnibus Budget Reconciliation Act (COBRA) insurance policy for eighteen months, and have elected not to purchase insurance because of the cost. These particular folks are hoping that they can remain healthy for the remaining years until they qualify for Medicare. Sure, they may have been fairly healthy and believe this is a calculated risk, and they do have a little money set aside if they need to pay cash for some minor medical expenses that could arise.

The projected numbers suggest that 18 million of the 34 million people who are not insured will now qualify for Medicaid under the PPACA. That's because the PPACA expands the eligibility requirements significantly to 133 percent of the federal poverty guideline.[1] The federal poverty guideline for 2011 is $22,050 for a family of four and $10,830 for an individual. Therefore, the eligibility requirements for Medicaid now mean that if you have a family of four and you make $29,326 or less, or if you are an individual and you now make $14,403, then you now qualify to receive Medicaid benefits as your health insurance.[2]

That sounds fine and dandy if you are currently uninsured. But let's talk about the reality of Medicaid. What is this government program's reputation within the medical community and the current patients who receive Medicaid? Basically, it's an inefficient and an ineffective program that is detested by both doctors and patients alike. When I was in family medicine, there were few things more frustrating in my daily duties than having to deal with the folks at Medicaid. It quickly became clear to me with every call to Medicaid that the main objective was to NOT pay for the medical service. If a patient on Medicaid needed a CT scan, we had to jump through all kinds of hoops before this service was paid for. And worse yet, if we happened to fail to get approval for the study before actually performing the service, it was classified as physician or administrative error, and no one got paid.

One of the most irritating things of all regarding Medicaid and Medicare is that if you, as a doctor or health care provider, agree to be a participant (i.e., you agree to accept Medicaid patients), then the government requires you to accept whatever payment they decide to give for the services rendered. For example, I am an FP and a patient comes to see me with an earache. My routine charge for an office visit is $35. If Medicaid has determined that they will pay only $17.50 for this level of office visit, then that is what I must accept. I cannot bill the patient for the remaining $17.50. When doctors or clinicians agree to be in-network providers, meaning that they agree to take Medicaid patients, it is made crystal clear when they sign the forms to be providers that they WILL accept the fees that Medicaid has assigned for each service. Attempting to collect the remainder of the office fee is considered illegal. The media and the PPACA supporters commonly note how much abuse and fraud there is in Medicaid and Medicare, but attempting to collect the total fee is one of the loose examples that they have incorrectly labeled as fraud and abuse.

If your grocery store bill is $35 and you have $17.50 in food stamps (now known as the Supplemental Nutrition Assistance Program, or SNAP), the grocer is not required to accept the food stamps and waive the additional $17.50 that you owe for your purchase. But in health care, we are expected to take this loss. And now, the government and the PPACA are expanding the Medicaid roles by an expected 18 million people. Do you think that doctors are pleased about this? This means we will have to see even more patients, get paid less per patient, or opt out of the system. I suspect there will be an exodus of participants from the Medicaid program from the health providers' standpoint. Government officials have predicted this and are proposing a fine for doctors if they leave Medicaid. There is also some discussion about mandating or requiring doctors to accept Medicaid and Medicare patients.

Have you ever thought about winning the lottery or Publishers Clearing House sweepstakes? Just pondering what it would be like causes some internal intrigue or excitement. Government officials are treating Medicaid with the same enthusiasm. To solve much of our uninsured woes, you, too, can now be on Medicaid. Well, the truth is, that's not such a great deal.

MEDICAID

Let's briefly look at how Medicaid works, or perhaps works ineffectively would be more accurate. Medicaid was signed into law in 1965 as a means of providing health care for our impoverished citizens, the poor among us. The program is overseen by the federal government, but it's implemented and administered at the state level. Each state is granted the leeway to design and implement the program in the manner that it sees fit. In 2008, Medicaid covered 43 million people, or 14 percent of the population. Under the PPACA, Medicaid will expand to nearly 60 million citizens with a price tag of about $410 billion, according to their own CMS numbers.[3] In 2008, the federal government paid for $204 billion or 57 percent of Medicaid expenses.[4]

In 2008, more Americans were on Medicaid (43 million) than were considered at or below the poverty guideline (39.1 million). Remember, the PPACA mandates that states will now include anyone who earns up to 133 percent of the federal poverty guideline. We are taking an inefficient program and expanding the number of people who will be receiving Medicaid. This requirement starts in 2014. Yet, the taxes we will discuss in a later chapter began in 2010.[5] You may say that putting the money away early to fund this is a good idea. Well, consider this: When the government and the media attempt to convince the American people that the PPACA is affordable, they use some fuzzy math. They began calculating the expense of the program in 2010, when the taxes took effect, and they discuss the first ten years until 2020. What they should do is calculate the expense based on when the actual insurance plan begins in 2014 and then the next ten years until 2024. However, here's the reason they don't show you the real expense numbers: The CBO expects the cost of the plan from 2014 through 2024 to be $2.5 trillion instead of $938 billion (the expected price from 2010 to 2020).[6] As usual, when Congress has an agenda—like forcing health care reform on the American people—they have an uncanny way of being deceptive or distorting the facts. In my opinion, this is shameful.

So, how is Medicaid doing? I think you'll be shocked at just how ineffective this program really is. Typically, a doctor receives around $200 for an hour-long consultation with a privately insured patient.[7] Did you know that doctors in New York generally earn $20 for a consultation with an established Medicaid patient? And this isn't exclusive to New York; this is the norm in every state. You couldn't get your front lawn mowed for that, nor could you get a plumber to come to your house for five times that amount. If the doctor misses a diagnosis, he or she assumes the liability. Most doctors lose money with every Medicaid patient they see. They also spend hours filling out the unbelievable number of form pages that are a part of the thousands of regulations the federal government places on the Medicaid system.

In most states, Medicaid is one of the three most expensive programs. On average, each state spends 22 percent on Medicaid.[8] In 2008, California spent $38.3 billion on Medi-Cal, California's Medicaid system. This included $25.6 billion from the federal government and $12.7 billion from the state of California. This was the highest amount in the nation. And California, like many of our states, is facing huge budget deficits. Many states are essentially bankrupt[9] because governors have followed Congress's example and have overspent their own treasuries to the point of bankruptcy. The PPACA will be expanding the number of people on Medicaid (most experts believe the number of Medicaid recipients will double), but the program is ineffective and already financially overspent; it is broke. Who is going to pay for this? You can't continue to cut payments to doctors and to hospitals without a complete collapse of the entire system.

Doctors are leaving the Medicaid system in droves. Why wouldn't they? Why should the doctors continue to see the Medicaid patient while taking a loss at the same time? When you take into consideration all the overhead expenses associated with a medical practice, $20 per consultation doesn't begin to pay the bills. From 200 to 2010, the number of Texas physicians participating in Medicaid decreased from 67 percent to 42 percent.[10] This is the trend all over the country.

MEDICAID ABUSE

Then there's the problem with overuse of the emergency department. Medicaid patients are also frustrated with the system. With the decreasing number of physicians accepting Medicaid patients, it's harder for Medicaid recipients to find a PCP. So, to have their medical needs met, they have universally turned to the emergency department and to hospitals for their immediate medical care, regardless of whether their ailment would be classified as emergent. In 2010, the Centers for Disease Control and Prevention (CDC) reported that more than 30 percent of patients aged sixty-five and under had visited an emergency department for medical care. Conversely, in 2007, fewer than 20 percent of patients with private insurance had sought care from their emergency department.[11]

Hospitals have a more difficult time than doctors in opting out of Medicaid. Like physician practices, hospitals are also receiving bare-bone reimbursement for the treatment and services rendered to Medicaid patients at their facilities. Often, the amount of reimbursement for the emergency treatment given to the Medicaid patient is less than the cost of delivering the care to begin with. According to the CBO, the total underpayments to hospitals from Medicaid for the medical treatment they rendered was $3.8 billion in 2000 and rose to $32 billion in 2008,[12] with no end to this shortfall in sight. In what other profession do we, as a society, expect the individual, institution, or company to take a loss in order to provide the services mandated by the government? There isn't any other profession like this.

In short, expanding Medicaid is not a solution. In fact, it's exactly the opposite: It compounds the problem. Medicaid delivers poor, inefficient, and slow service. It's loaded with abuse and fraud and is saddled with extensive regulations. No, fellow citizens, the answer to the health care woes does not lie with the expansion of Medicaid. Our president, Congress, and the media realize this. But it isn't really about finding reasonable and responsible solutions to our health delivery system; rather, it's more about growing a bigger government that gains more control of all our lives, decreases our choices and our freedoms, and ultimately forces every one of us into a single-payer system. When this happens, we will have become a completely socialistic country rather than a republic. From all indications, this isn't too far away!

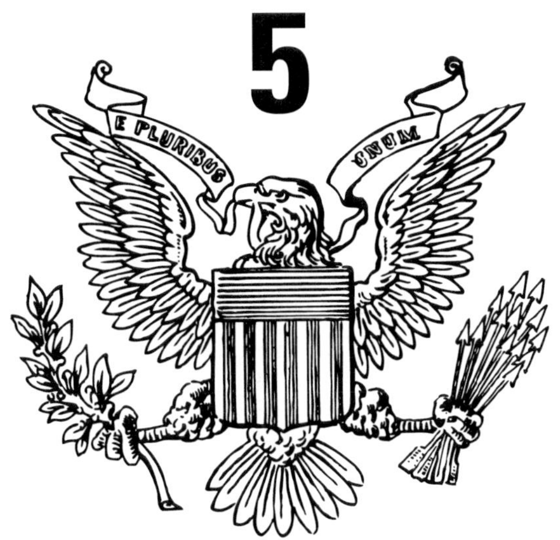

5

MANDATE

The online Free Dictionary by Farlex (www.thefreediction-ary.com) defines *mandate* as "an authoritative command or instruction" or "to make mandatory, as by law; decree or require."[1] Within the health care reform bill, there are numerous instructions or commands. Specifically, let's look at the law or requirement to purchase health insurance. There are two categories of mandate regarding purchasing health insurance: the individual mandate and the employer mandate. Within the PPACA is the requirement (not the request or suggestion) that every citizen of the United States MUST purchase health insurance or face an annual fine. The media and the current administration will tell you that there is no employer mandate included in the PPACA, and, technically, this could be construed as true. However, here's what it says within the bill: Employers with more than fifty employees MUST provide health insurance for their employees or pay a fine.

Many questions arise regarding these mandates. Are there any exceptions? If so, who? How will this be enforced? What are the fines or penalties? When does this go into effect? Will you still be able to choose your insurance company and the policy that best meets your needs? Will you still be allowed to select the physician or provider you desire?

But even before these questions are answered, there is a more fundamental issue to discuss, namely, whether the federal government has any right to mandate anything to the American people. Is placing this demand on its citizens in accordance with the Constitution? Since the bill's passage on March 23, 2010, the constitutionality of this mandate has been questioned. According to the Independent Association of Businesses, there are now twenty-five states suing regarding the constitutionality of the mandate requiring all citizens to purchase health insurance.[2] The debate over this topic suggests that if the mandate is ultimately determined unconstitutional, then the entire PPACA legislation should be considered null and void. This lawsuit will probably end up in the hands of the US Supreme Court. However, even if the Court were to deem this mandate unconstitutional, don't believe for one minute that it will mark the end of the PPACA. First, it's quite unlikely that the highest court in the land will determine the mandate unconstitutional; the highest probability I've seen of this happening is 25 percent, which means there's a three-in-four chance it will be determined legal and acceptable pertaining to our constitutional rights. Second, even if the Court did surprise America and say the government has over stepped its boundaries, that will not be the end of the PPACA, even if logically it appears that it should be. Likely, Congress will amend the current law—remember, it has already passed both houses of Congress and has been signed into law,[3] and we already have well over a year of groundwork laid to implement this monstrosity of legislation. Congress would probably change the law from a requirement or mandate[4] to a suggestion that, if not complied with, would lead to increases in our current taxes. Congress is *H_-bent* on making this health reform legislation happen.

Interestingly, there is one other possibility with regards to the constitutionality of the PPCACA, and it is known as the severability clause. In the house version of the PPACA, there was severability language included in the bill. However, this clause did not make it into the Senate version, which ultimately became law. Exclusion of the severability clause means, basically, is that if any bill is determined to be unconstitutional, then, in the absence of the severability clause, the entire bill is automatically concluded to be unconstitutional, on the merit of solitary unconstitutional element. Or, another way of saying this, if a single portion of the bill is determined by the courts to be unconstitutional, then the entire bill is unconstitutional based on that single item, and the entire bill is scrapped. Whereas, in the presence of the severability clause, if a single item is unconstitutional, that one item is excluded, but the remainder of the bill remains.

CONSTITUTIONALITY

Is the bill constitutional? Does Congress have this right to make these demands of American citizens? Congress says they absolutely have this authority and power because of the Commerce Clause in the Constitution. This clause grants Congress the power to regulate commerce. To try to determine who is correct, let's turn to a legal authority and get his opinion. In his March 2010 *Washington Post* article titled "Is Health-Care Reform Constitutional?,"[5] Randy Barnett, JD, Carmack Waterhouse Professor of Legal Theory at the Georgetown University Law Center, suggested Congress is taking some significant liberties with the purpose of the Commerce Clause, which is unprecedented. Congress has never before used its commerce power to mandate that an individual engage in an economic transaction with a private company.[6] Not even during World War II did Congress mandate that individual citizens purchase war bonds (even though purchasing these bonds was for the overall good and well-being of the country). That's the point: In a republic, the government does NOT tell their citizens what they must purchase or how they shall go about purchasing whatever it is the government officials are suggesting. Congress has overstepped its authority by penalizing or fining citizens who do not comply. Hence, twenty-five states have entered into a legal battle with the federal government, questioning the constitutionality of the mandate and ultimately the entire PPACA.

One other interesting tidbit regarding this mandate: You may recall that Barack Obama campaigned against this in 2008 when he was running for president. Aren't you amazed at how quickly politicians change their stance on major issues? Ask yourself how many times you jump from one side of an issue to another. At a certain age in our adulthood, most of us reach the place where we have a pretty good idea where we stand or how certain we feel about most major societal and political issues. Sure, we always reserve the right to change our mind or to be convinced of the opposite side of any issue, but it doesn't happen too frequently. It's called knowing where you stand and having conviction for what you believe. Yet, politicians seem to change from one side of an issue to the other, almost as often as they change their clothes, depending on the political expedience.

WHY NOT OPT OUT?

Now, what if you choose not to accept this individual mandate, and you refuse to purchase health insurance? What if you are one of the uninsured currently in America, and you electively choose to thumb your nose at Congress? What are the repercussions? Those who ignore the mandate to purchase health insurance will pay the following fine or penalty, starting in 2014: The noncompliance will cost $695, or 2.5 percent of a person's household income up to a total fine of $2,085, whichever is higher. Remember, the folks who are 133 percent the federal poverty guideline have already been placed on Medicaid.[7] An employer with fifty or more employees will be required to provide health insurance to those employees or pay a fine of $2,000 per worker.

ANY EXEMPTIONS?

Is anyone exempt from this mandate? Yes, and it may surprise you just which groups of people are exempt. Christian Scientists (who do not adhere to orthodox medical treatment), Scientologists, Native Americans, and Muslims (who apparently oppose insurance altogether) get a free pass.[8] Don't misunderstand me; I don't believe it is appropriate for Congress to place this mandate on any of the American people, but if the US Supreme Court upholds it, and it's determined that it will happen, could I declare that purchasing health insurance goes against my religious beliefs? Could I therefore be exempt, too, as a conscientious objector? If it's deemed constitutional and the bill stands as is, is it appropriate or fair to exempt any one of our citizens from this mandate?

Then there's the logical question: If the health insurance plan costs, say, $300 per month for an individual or $3,600 per year, and the penalty is only $695 per year for not having insurance, wouldn't any logical and financially savvy individual elect to accept the fine or the penalty rather than purchase the insurance policy? So, the only way that a mandate works is if the punishment for not purchasing the required product (health insurance, in this case) is more painful than not purchasing the product. Under the current rules of the PPACA, that is not the case. Citizens will elect not to purchase health insurance because the penalty will cost significantly less than the policy itself. Then what is different about this requirement from what we currently face? There will still remain a significant number of citizens who choose to pay the fine and not purchase health insurance. Of course, at least a total of $695 per year per uninsured person will go towards paying for the PPACA . The natural conclusion will be that Congress, over time, will impose greater fines and penalties until it becomes too costly to not purchase the health insurance policy. So much for our personal choices and freedoms!

UNINSURED

Throughout the health care debate during the entire year of 2009, it was stated over and over that there are 46.3 million Americans (including 8 million children) who are without health insurance. Depending on what source you refer to, the number has been reported as low as 34 million and as high as 50 million. But, because the most frequently quoted number has been 46.3 million, let's use this number, which comes from the US Census Bureau. This amounts to 15.4 percent of our population.[9]

Who are these uninsured Americans? The media would have you believe that these uninsured citizens are the poorest among us who can't afford to buy health insurance. Well, this idea that they are the poorest of our society couldn't be further from the truth. Of the 46.3 million uninsured, 9.7 million make more than $75,000 a year.[10] Good, you say. They can afford to buy health insurance. Another 14 million of the 46.3 million Americans are eligible for Medicare, Medicaid, or the State Children's Health Insurance Program (SCHIP); however, they have elected not to enroll. Of the 46.3 million, 6 million qualify for employer-sponsored insurance but have elected not to participate. Another 5 million are recent immigrants who have just become US citizens; as crazy as it may sound, 5.2 million illegal immigrants were included in the 46.3 million total.[11] So, when you add up all these numbers, there are actually about 6.4 million Americans who lack affordable health insurance. This number sounds much less ominous or at least much more manageable than the commonly stated 46.3 million.

Why would these 9.7 million Americans who make $75,000 or more a year choose not to purchase health insurance, and is it really any of our business? If they expect a free ride from Joe Taxpayer, then of course it's our business. But if they are paying cash for their health care, because they can, then what difference should it make to any of us whether they choose to purchase health insurance? It's been said that this number is actually a snapshot of the uninsured; many of these folks aren't chronically uninsured. In other words, these folks may be between jobs or have chosen not to pay the COBRA policy during periods of job change or relocation, or these folks may have elected to forgo health insurance for a few months for financial reasons. They may feel that they can afford to pay cash if, by chance, they happen to need any medical care over a period of a few months rather than pay for an expensive policy. And if these people are under the age of forty or forty-five, this could make some financial sense. After all, if they are generally healthy, the odds that they will be able to afford the minimal (if any) care that they need may be a calculated risk they are willing to take. Again, if they are productive members of society, and if they are tax-paying citizens who pay their own way, why should I care if they choose not to purchase health insurance or if they choose not to seek routine medical attention? This certainly wouldn't work for everyone, especially the middle age and elderly, because it would be highly risky However, it may actually be financially sound for some.

If you add up all the numbers of each defined group, the total is greater than 46.3 million. How can that be? Well, some of the individuals qualify for more than one group. For example, of the $75,000-annual-income crowd, some of these folks may also be included in the 6 million people of the employer-sponsored group who have elected not to use the employer-sponsored health insurance. Taking this overlap into consideration, there's an additional group of 8 million of these 46.3 million who reportedly make an annual income between $50,000 and $74,999. If you add this group to the $75,000-plus group of 9.7 million people, that makes a total of 17.7 million of the 46.3 million,[12] which means that 38.2 percent of this 46.3 million who have chosen, for whatever reason, not to purchase health insurance are certainly not members of the impoverished class of citizens, as Congress and the media would lead you to believe! Once again, Congress and our media distort and withhold all the information to fulfill their own agenda.

Of course, there's the largest pool of uninsured known as the invincible crowd. They are between the ages of 20-35 years and believe they won't get sick. It's a calculated risk but certainly one they should have the right to make themselves, especially if they are willing to accept the natural consequences, if they should fall ill.

I'm more concerned about the 14 million Americans who already qualify for Medicaid, Medicare, or SCHIP but have elected not to sign up. Regardless of their reason for not signing up for this subsidy, their unwillingness to participate has contributed to the overall perception that health care is truly in crisis. I've already admitted that the current system has some problems, and I will address some reasonable solutions in a later chapter. But the one universally stated reason for venturing into the health care reform debate was that we have 34 to 50 million Americans who are uninsured. The implication or inference is that somehow these poor citizens had been overlooked or left out, and that just isn't the case. So, Congress, using misleading numbers, raised enough public concern that they managed to force the PPACA through Congress. Now we are dealing with a massive change in a so-called failing system to help all these uninsured people when the premise that there are 34 to 50 million people without insurance was flawed and misleading from the beginning. These inaccurate and misleading numbers have enabled a societal debate and ultimate outcome of complete overhaul of an existing health system that has some problems but really only needed some tweaking, not a complete makeover or remake.

WORKING UNINSURED

Then there's the illegal immigrant crowd. Why is this group even included in the number of uninsured American citizens if they aren't even legal citizens of the United States? Send them home, or enforce steps toward legal immigration. Of course, as ridiculous as it sounds, some of these illegal immigrants are receiving health benefits. This is specifically true for the illegal immigrant's newborn child who is fortunate enough to be born in one of our American hospitals. This newborn infant is automatically a US citizen.[13] If my wife and I were illegal immigrants in any foreign country, and if she gave birth to our child in that country, do you suppose our child would automatically be considered a full-fledged citizen of that country? I don't think so! Only in America!

There is the legitimate group of uninsured individuals who make less than $50,000 a year and who work hard to pay their bills.[14] They are productive, hard-working, proud Americans who simply cannot afford the rising health care premiums. These truly are the uninsured whom we should be speaking about, for the current system has truly failed them. Here is where we should have been focusing our real attention. This is one of the real problems that exist with our current system, and here is where we should have been tweaking the system to provide some reasonable solutions for this group of citizens. These people would benefit from an affordable catastrophic health insurance plan. They also may be able to afford a basic level-of-care plan. For example, for a reasonable premium, these individuals above the federal poverty guideline but earning less than $50,000 could benefit from a plan that offered basic preventive care up to $5,000 or $10,000 a year or catastrophes above $50,000. This type of a plan would assist these folks and provide them the type of real reform that they are looking for. Instead, we ignore even discussing these types of solutions and go straight to a complete overhaul of the existing system, under the pretense that about 15 percent of our population is unable to purchase health insurance.

What happens if you don't purchase health insurance? What if you dare the government to fine you? Will the government actually collect these fines, and, if so, how will they go about taking your hard-earned money? Who will be the oversight organization to collect these fees? The answer is the IRS. Currently, the IRS is adding between 16,000 and 16,500 IRS agents whose job description includes seeing that all Americans participate in the PPACA and comply with the mandate of purchasing insurance. These agents will ensure that fines are given to individuals if they do not purchase health insurance for themselves and to businesses with fifty or more employees[15] if they do not purchase health insurance for their workers. How will they go about collecting the penalties? Currently, they cannot go into your bank account and confiscate your money, put a lien on your assets until you pay, or garnish your wages. Instead, they are allowed (and intend) to reduce or eliminate your tax refunds. When it comes to confiscating your hard-earned money, those in the government always find a way!

6

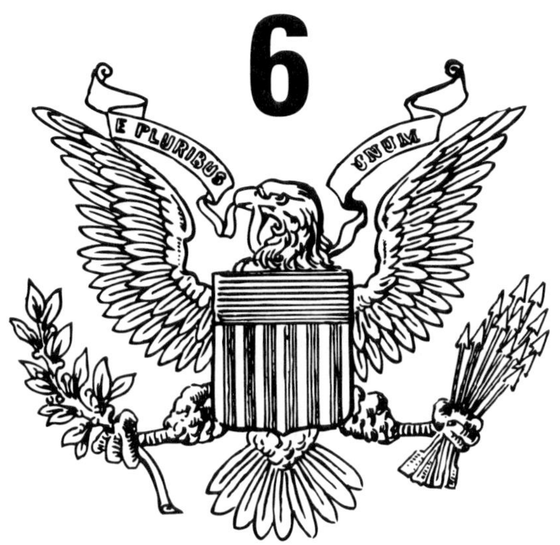

LET'S GET TO THE DETAILS.

For some reason, it was extremely important for the supporters of the Patient Protection and Affordable Care Act to include the requirement that no child is left off his or her parent's health insurance plan eligibility. If I asked you at what age a child becomes an adult in this country, what would be your response? Is it sixteen, eighteen, or twenty-one years? Or, perhaps a reasonable answer would be when the child finishes an undergraduate education at age twenty-two. Would anyone answer with twenty-six years? Under the PPACA, insurance companies must allow children to stay on their parents' health insurance plan until age twenty-six.[1]

In America, according to the Constitution, you can be elected to the US House of Representatives at age twenty-five.[2] Can you picture a twenty-five-year-old being elected to the House, contracting a medical malady, and having to request his mother to send a facsimile of her insurance card to the hospital emergency department so that he can receive treatment? Isn't that absurd?

It's so ridiculous that it must be true, as no one could make up something so foolish. The adage "truth is stranger than fiction" is absolutely true in this instance!

PREEXISTING CONDITIONS

Another extremely important tenet of the PPACA is to prevent insurance companies from denying coverage to children because of a preexisting condition. This went into effect six months after the bill's passage in September 2010. In 2014, insurance companies cannot deny insurance coverage to adults with a preexisting condition. This has received a great deal of attention with the media. It even sounds like a reasonable requirement. However, there are a couple of items we need to discuss to really grasp the full impact of this requirement. What many people don't realize is that cancelling insurance based on preexisting conditions has been illegal in this country for the past decade. What has made this somewhat complicated is that many of us have heard horror stories about people having their insurance policies cancelled. We have even heard of cases in which patients have developed some serious illness and insurance companies have refused to pay for their medical care or they discontinued the policies. Each specific case must be looked at individually.

It is true that an insurance company cannot cancel your policy for any reason, unless you quit paying your premiums or unless you lie on your application. Both these reasons are grounds for termination.[3] Now, that doesn't mean that the premiums couldn't go up. This has been a tactic that many health insurance companies have used over the years. If a person develops an unusual medical condition—let's say something very rare like systemic lupus erythematosus, a rare connective tissue disorder where your skin and your tissues begin to harden throughout your body—it is feasible that the insurance company could increase your premiums to the point where they are no longer affordable. The insurance company could also deny certain therapies, treatments, surgeries, or medications because of your particular coverage. Or, it could even say it will pay for specific treatments up to a certain dollar amount or up to a certain cap. But to flat out cancel a policy is illegal and has been since 2000. To claim to the American people that they now cannot have their policy cancelled is a bit disingenuous, for it couldn't happen with their current private insurance. Also, do you think that the federal government will give all people unlimited health care under the PPACA? If so, then you are extremely naïve or gullible. The current administration states unequivocally that Americans will not have rationed care. Yet, the same administration has often admitted that there will be decisions based on cost and cost containment. This is code for "rationed health care" or "limited health services." There isn't any way around this. The cost of unlimited health care for all people is and has always been more expensive than America has the resources to pay for it. One of the regulations that the media and much of America are applauding is the forbidding of private or public insurance from cancelling individual policies based on preexisting conditions—but this is nothing new. We are an uninformed people much of the time! Having said that, I understand why we are uninformed. With all the confusing and contradictory information out there, who knows what is true and what isn't?

Turn to your own personal experiences or the experiences of your friends and family for many of the answers. For example, if your uncle lost his job, didn't he also lose his insurance? He may have technically lost his current insurance policy, but he was probably given the opportunity to purchase a COBRA policy that was effective for eighteen months after he lost his job and his current policy was discontinued. If he was capable of paying for the eighteen months of the COBRA policy, and if he was able to gain employment with health insurance coverage and maintained continual coverage without any gaps, then the insurance company could not deny him coverage for any existing, new, or preexisting condition.[4]

Granted, it's true that COBRA policies are more expensive, and there are some very specific and even rigid requirements that a person must meet to maintain continual health insurance coverage. Therefore, it is reasonable to take a long, hard look at these current limitations, regulations, and restrictions and determine if there isn't a better way to deal with these particular situations that do arise regarding loss of employment and health care coverage and preexisting conditions. But, once again, instead of closely studying the current system, recognizing its shortcomings, and trying to correct the problems and improve an otherwise pretty good health care system, we scrap the current system and start over with a brand new program that is wrought with even greater problems, some of which have yet to even be identified!

A story by Kathleen Parker in the July 19, 2011 edition of the *Topeka Capital Journal* recalled how President Obama told the story of his mother's fight with uterine and ovarian cancer at age fifty-two.[5] During the 2008 presidential race, the then-senator Obama recalled on more than one occasion how his mother, Ann Dunham, fought the insurance companies to pay for her cancer treatment. "I will never forget my own mother, as she fought cancer in her final months, having to worry about whether her insurance would refuse to pay for her treatment." He described how his mother fought until her dying breath with an uncaring insurance company about payments for her cancer treatment. According to Senator Obama, the company wouldn't pay because his mother's cancer was considered a preexisting condition.

One of the central components of the PPACA health reform bill is the desire to eliminate preexisting conditions as an obstacle to insurance coverage. Senator Obama's story was used to touch the hearts of a sympathetic nation. Its portrayal of corporate insurance's inhumanity toward his mother's preexisting condition became a key component in convincing a willing public. The only problem is that the story was not true. In her book *A Singular Woman: The Untold Story of Barrack Obama's Mother*, Janny Scott says that Ann Dunham's cancer treatments were covered by her employer's insurance policy. Apparently, she was denied disability insurance, but her cancer treatments were never denied. When the White House was questioned regarding this account in Ms. Scott's book, they declined to refute its validity. Their only explanation was that the president told the story about his mother based on his recollection of events that took place more than fifteen years ago.

This personal recollection became Senator Obama's most compelling argument for health reform. In her story that ran in the *Topeka Capital Journal*, Kathleen Parker asked, "Is it too much to say that Obama told an intentionally tall tale to mislead the public?" But it is also incorrect to say that he told a true story. He intentionally used this personal anecdote to make his argument for health care reform. It's concerning that a bigger agenda can cloud one's memory. Did this omission persuade America to stop the uncaring corporate world of insurance from doing even more damage? The polls still suggest that America didn't want the PPACA[6] then, and they still don't now." So, Senator Obama's story wasn't as persuasive as he had probably hoped. What is more distressing is that a personal story of this magnitude could be slightly twisted to accomplish one's political agenda. It points to the willingness and audacity to use any and all means to accomplish a political goal.

Why can't all our politicians and the supporters and creators of the PPACA be forthright with the American people? I believe it's because they have a bigger agenda than providing quality health care to the American people; I believe it's ultimately to create a single-payer system in which private insurance and insurance options are obsolete. I think they want each of us on a government-run health insurance program—except for Christian Scientists, Scientologists, Native Americans, probably Congress (I suspect they will exempt themselves from such a government-run program and provide themselves with unlimited cart blanche medical care, for at least that's their normal pattern of behavior with other benefits to themselves), and of course Muslims!

7

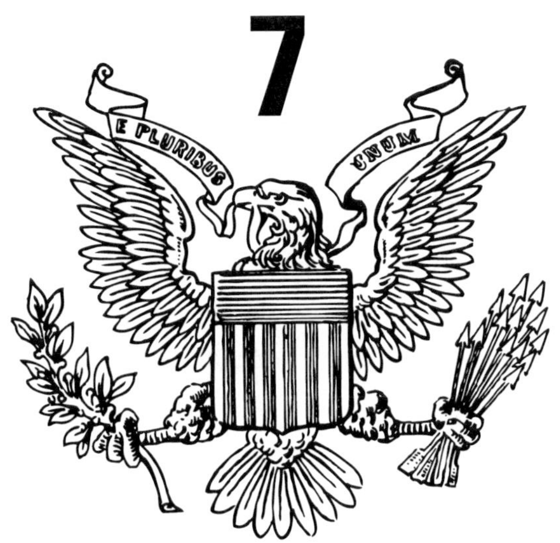

MORE MANDATES

Earlier I stated that the PPACA includes two mandates. The first one is that all American citizens (except Christian Scientists, Scientologists, Native Americans, Muslims, and apparently members of Congress) are required to purchase health insurance. The second mandate is the employer mandate requiring all American companies with fifty or more employees to provide health insurance for their workers. If these two mandates are not met, then the individuals and companies are given a fine. Besides these two obvious mandates, there are other specific mandates or requirements, too. Let's take a look at some of the more specific insurance policy requirements, which I will refer to as benefits or mandates.

CURRENT INSURANCE REQUIREMENTS

But first, let's take a look at the history of insurance requirements prior to the PPACA to gain a greater appreciation of the detailed expectations already placed on insurance companies. Government regulations dictating which services are or are not included in health policies have been around for decades before the PPACA even existed. In 1979, 252 state mandates were in place across the entire country, with an average of five requirements per state. By 2009, there were a total of 2,133 state mandates, or an average of forty-two per state.[1] These mandates were described on each health policy as benefits. Each state determined which individual mandate (or so-called benefit) must be included in each policy.

The mandates or benefits varied from state to state. Such requirements included covering hearing aids, paying for massage therapy services, dietician counseling or one-on-one nutritional counseling for people with morbid obesity (regardless of their current weight), hormone replacement surgery, or breast reduction surgery. How many average American citizens will ever have a need to consider breast reduction surgery? Regardless, in many states such surgery is a requirement for health insurance policies. Some states require alternative-medicine therapies like acupuncture, some require covering contraceptives, and others even require covering personal athletic trainers.

Most of the various state mandates or benefits in the right situation can be an excellent benefit for any one particular medical condition. But to require these numerous services for every state health insurance policy as a one-size-fits-all insurance plan is excessive and drives up the cost of insurance. Why would any state decide that any one particular service is so important that it is included as a state health insurance requirement or mandate? What makes any particular medical treatment more worthy of coverage than any other? This can be answered in one word: lobbyist. Special-interest groups such as chiropractors, massage therapists, or athletic trainers send their lobbyists to the state politicians and persuade the lawmakers to include their services on the state list of required health insurance benefits.

The Council of Economic Advisers looked at the overall effects of state health insurance requirements on the individual health policies. They determined that every individual health insurance mandate or requirement raises the overall price by 0.4 percent for individual policies and 0.5 percent for family policies.[2] Other organizations such as the Council for Affordable Health Insurance have reported that state mandates or requirements have the potential to increase health premiums by as much as 50 percent.[3] Most often, these increases in your health policy are for benefits that you will probably not use or need for your particular health care. Once again, why should we all pay for the benefits of others? Why couldn't each insurance plan be tailored to each individual's needs? Here is yet another example of how government officials decide what you must purchase, with the end result being more expensive for you. It would sure be a lot easier if the government would simply get out of the health insurance business and quit mandating the various health services.

PREVENTATIVE SERVICES

If these state mandates in our current health insurance policies have already resulted in increased costs, then what other mandates are included in the PPACA? Those of us in medicine have often suggested that Americans need to shift their focus from reactive medical care to proactive medical care; in other words, they should direct their attention to preventive medicine. Specifically, for example, women should schedule routine yearly mammograms and yearly breast exams starting at age forty rather than wait for a lump to develop at age forty-five and then race to their doctor. Now, if you have just developed a lump in your breast and you are reading this book, ignore what I just suggested and run straight to your doctor. But, if you haven't been complying with the recommendations regarding your breast exams and mammograms, then get started now or at age forty as suggested.

We've done a better job concentrating on some preventive services in America (e.g., screening mammograms). We have seen a steady decrease in breast cancer rates over the past decade because of our emphasis on women's health and mammography. According to breastcancer.org, the incidence of breast cancer in America has decreased by 2 percent per year, a significant reduction.[4] This is proof that we see positive results when we focus our attention on prevention. There's a reason the adage "an ounce of prevention is worth a pound of cure" is accurate.

In the PPACA, all insurance companies are mandated to cover preventive care in its entirety.[5] This sounds like a good idea, right? I agree; from a medical standpoint, this is where we should be placing our efforts. Well, what preventive measures are we referring to? All of them! Nearly anything you can come up with that is preventive must be covered by your current insurance company and definitely by the health insurance exchanges, which we will discuss in detail in an upcoming chapter. Let's take a look at some of these services: maternity and childcare (What if you're single and don't have any children?), substance abuse and rehabilitation services (What if you don't drink alcohol or use drugs?), Pap smears (What if you're not sexually active?), prostatic-specific antigen and digit rectal exam (What if you're a single female?), just to name a few. These common preventive services should be covered in your current health plan, and more than likely they already are. But each individual policy should be tailored to each individual's specific situation and specific needs. One size does not fit all! When you force everyone into the same plan with the same benefits, all it does is lead to increased costs. Do you think insurance companies or our government exchanges will eat these costs? They will not; they'll pass this on to the consumer in the form of increased premiums. So much for the continued promise that if you like your current policy and you want to keep it, your current premiums will not go up. There's no way around this. If the government mandates a large list of benefits to be included in each health plan, then the only logical conclusion is that your premiums will go up.

How many of these mandates should we expect? As I stated earlier, from 1979 until 2009, the number of required state benefits grew from 252 to 2,133.[6] The exponential growth over thirty years was significant. Imagine what the exponential growth will be now that the federal government is involved in identifying and assigning these specific mandates. Their track record shows they overregulate anything they get their hands on. Even though they pay lip service to us that they will be frugal and practice financial responsibility, they do not. They have not shown the ability to be responsible with other people's money in any of their endeavors. That's why our deficit is over $13 trillion.[7] Do NOT believe them when they say your premiums will go down.

What about the benefit of focusing on preventive care? Currently, health insurance companies have done a much more thorough job of including and taking a closer look at providing preventive services for their clients. That doesn't mean there isn't room for improvement in this arena. However, if the government would step out of the way, the private sector would be able to solve these problems. Instead, Congress proceeds to scrap the current health system and start over with a whole new 2,562 page legislative nightmare, the PPACA.

8

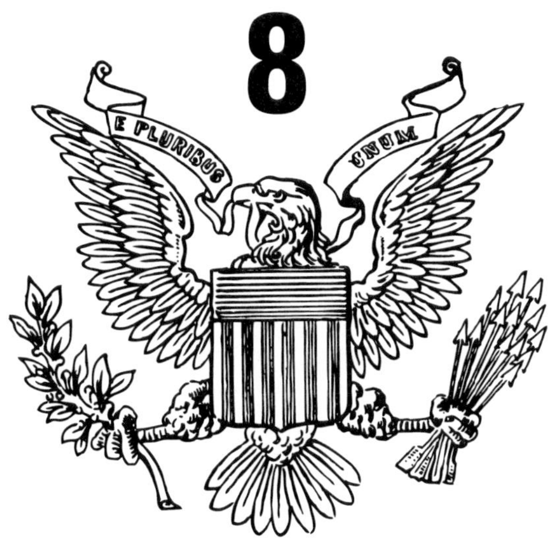

HEALTH EXCHANGES

The US House of Representatives had their own version of the health reform bill before the creation and passage of the PPACA, and in that version they included a solitary national exchange run by the HHS.[1] This version was changed to its current form, the PPACA, where it says the uninsured and self-employed would be able to purchase insurance through state-based exchanges with subsidies available to individuals and families with income between 133 percent and 400 percent[2] of the federal poverty guideline. Effective in 2014, separate exchanges would be created for small businesses to purchase coverage. Oversight of the exchanges shifted from another federal agency to individual state administration. Funding will be available to each state to establish these exchanges up to 2015.

HISTORY OF HEALTH EXCHANGES

Let's take a close look at these exchanges. The idea of health exchanges is nothing new. Congress established the Federal Employees Health Benefits (FEHB) program in 1959 to provide health insurance to federal employees and their families.[3] Instead of offering only a single health plan, the FEHB offered several different, but similar, health plans. Each of these plans was evaluated by the US Office of Personnel Management to confirm that they included each of the required mandates. This system gave the government workers an opportunity to have, or at least to feel as if they were given, free choice. Each of these plans was similar and included the requirements and benefits mandated by the federal government; however, each was dissimilar enough that the premiums were slightly different and the federal employees gained a sense of fairness and choice. But, in reality, the plans were more similar than dissimilar, and so the government was actually effectively managing the level of competition.

Bill Clinton's "Hillary" plan in the 1990s included a similar type of oversight and strict management of the various health insurance plans and their list of included benefits. Former president Clinton used the term "managed competition"[4] to try to sell this nationalized health plan to the American people, and the FEHB example from 1959 served as the model for these few government-managed health insurance plans.

King Solomon said, "There is nothing new under the sun,"[5] and the longer I live, the more I realize how wise he really was—at least regarding the US government, there is nothing new under the sun! Throughout his presidential campaign, Senator Obama's platform included the creation of a single, regulated marketplace for health insurance called a national health insurance exchange. In 2010, President Obama and his team of health policy wonks, with a similar agenda to each of these past administrations, coined the new phrase "health exchanges."[6] When you study these exchanges closely, you see a great similarity between the few health plans offered by the FEHB in 1959 and the managed competition that would oversee the health insurance policies in the 1990s. Another adage that accurately describes the federal government is that they are like a dog with a bone. Starting with Franklin Delano Roosevelt, the Democrats have insisted that they would gain total control over the health insurance system. Just like a dog who won't give up that juicy bone, the federal government latched onto the topic of health care for eighty years before getting their hands on all our health care bones.

EXCHANGE DETAILS

Each state will receive federal "start-up" money to create "American health insurance exchanges."[7] Each state is required to develop, recruit, manage, and regulate a variety of health insurance plans so that each of our uninsured citizens (minus those who now qualify for the expanded Medicaid ranks or those expanded pools of employees whose employers are now required to provide health insurance) will be able to evaluate and personally choose which policy he or she wants. It could look something like a marketplace or a shopping mall for insurance plans, managed by each individual state.

Another important caveat is determining whom these exchanges were developed for and how they will be affordable. A few of the current problems I've already discussed are people being unable to afford their own insurance plans, having employers who have chosen not to provide health insurance, or making too much money to qualify for assistance. These are generally the folks whose income falls between the federal poverty guideline and $50,000. Remember, with the PPACA, Medicaid will be expanded to include 133 percent of the 2011 federal poverty guideline, or $29,327 for a family of four. How do these exchanges help these folks who make between

$29,327 and $50,000?[8] They are already struggling to afford health insurance. Here's how: subsidies.

The PPACA will provide federal subsidies to those who make between 133 percent and 400 percent of the federal poverty guideline. A family of four, with two adults and two children, who make between $29,327 and $88,200 (400 percent above the federal poverty guideline) will receive a subsidy from the federal government. Talk about expanding our entitlement state! You can see why I have raised grave concerns about how we are allowing the federal government to grow even larger and how we will ultimately achieve complete socialization of our country. Everywhere we turn is expansion of our current entitlement state. An income of nearly $90,000 now entitles the income earner for a government entitlement, a subsidy, a handout. Is that unbelievable? It used to be that a $90,000 income was considered pretty good money. When did it change to the point that people with such an income now need assistance? Couldn't better management of their resources or their household budgets be a better answer rather than a handout? Oh, that's right; we have the federal and state governments as our example for money management. I guess an entitlement is the only answer for them!

Let's take a hypothetical look at a state-run exchange. Picture this: You and your family have fallen through the cracks. You make $52,000, but your self-employed employer only has six employees and has therefore elected not to pay for your health insurance. Your subsidy check (in theory) has arrived in the mail with a letter suggesting that you have health insurance by 2014 but requiring you have it by 2016. You head to your local strip mall that no longer has private businesses but instead has slowly and methodically become a state and federal government strip mall.

The boutique that used to be in the strip mall sold out to the state health insurance agency in 2011, and this is where you head to purchase your insurance.

When you arrive, the parking lot is packed, so you have to park two lots over. You choose to walk because you think the quarter-mile trek would do you some good. Halfway across the second lot, the shuttle passes by. It sure looks similar to an amusement park shuttle, but they should put some colorful animated caricatures on the side. You realize the fortune in your decision to walk because the shuttle is overflowing, with every seat taken and at least ten people standing. Then it dawns on you: All those people are being dropped at the door, which means your decision to walk might have cost you twenty or thirty places in line. So, you pick up your pace, hoping that most of these people are heading to the Division of Motor Vehicles (DMV), which is next door to the health insurance agency. This strip mall that was brand new in 2000 has become the location for the DMV; the Women, Infants, and Children and welfare offices; Social Security; and now the crown jewel, the state health insurance agency—home to the health exchange.

You're intrigued; you are interested to see what options are available to you and what they will cost. But you have been an independent and aren't sure if you support the government takeover of health insurance, yet you'll be glad to give it a try. When you walk through the door, you see a waiting area with at least fifty aluminum folding chairs, nothing fancy. For a second you have the déjà vu experience, then you realize this looks distinctly like the DMV. For a split second you recall your last trip to get your car tags and you cringe, for that experience took you three and a half hours.

A desk in the middle of the room is clearly marked as the information desk. You stand in line behind seven people. After ten minutes, it's your turn. That wasn't too bad, you tell yourself, and you hand the woman behind the desk your letter. "Oh, it's 10:15, and I have a break until 10:30. You can take a seat and I'll be right with you," she says as she abruptly leaves. Fifteen minutes later, she returns. You stayed at the front of the line to keep your place. She says, "Oh, you'll need to fill out these forms. Also, take a number, and when your number is called you will go to that window over there and you'll be ushered into the exchange."

You take number 211 and your packet of forms and have a seat. You begin filling out the questionnaire as you hear the clerk say "One-four-seven? Number one-four-seven." The packet includes an exhaustive health questionnaire for your entire family. You wonder if you couldn't get this from your current doctor and just ask him to give a copy of your family's medical history to whichever insurance company you choose.

About an hour later, the clerk says "Number two hundred." You look at your clock and see it's now 11:30. This worries you as you wonder what happens if your number is called at 11:59. Will they ask you to wait until 1:00 because of the mandated hour-long lunch break? Fortunately, the clerk calls your number at 11:45 and you enter the back room before lunch time. As you walk through the door, you notice a significant change in the atmosphere. In the waiting room you were seated in an aluminum folding chair on cement, and the room itself has drab gray walls. But when you enter the back room, you notice a hallway with five different offices. The floor is carpeted, pictures hang on the walls, and the furniture is of high quality. This is the work of a skilled interior decorator, you tell yourself.

BRONZE, SILVER, GOLD, PLATINUM

At the front of the hallway is a woman behind a desk. She asks for your questionnaire. After a couple of seconds she says, "I see that your husband has been infected with herpes simplex. I also see that you had cervical cancer. I think that puts you in the moderate-risk category. I also see that you make $52,000; that plus your subsidy qualifies you for a Silver or a Bronze policy. I suggest that you go to office number one or two." The personal nature of her comments about you and your husband's medical histories bothers you, and before you proceed to the first office you ask the woman, "Are you a nurse or a doctor?" She replies, "Are you kidding? I faint at the sight of blood." It dawns on you that this isn't your father's health care system. What happened to the Health Insurance Portability and Accountability Act (HIPAA) privacy laws?

The first office is labeled "Bronze" above the door. Upon entering the Bronze office, there are only two people in line in front of you. At noon, you are escorted into the back room. Behind yet another desk is yet another woman. She says, "Have a seat." You hand her your questionnaire and you have a seat.

"Do you have any questions?" she asks you.

You begin with the obvious: "What does 'Bronze' mean?"

She replies, "That's the least expensive policy we offer. There are four levels of plans: Bronze, Silver, Gold, and Platinum.[9] Looking at your income and your federal subsidy, it appears the Bronze will be the most affordable for you."

You ask her, "Does that mean my premiums with a Bronze plan would be less than, say, the Gold plan?"

She shakes her head. "Oh, no, all premiums are the same."

"So, why wouldn't I go straight to the Gold or Platinum plan?"

"Well," she explains, "those plans would cost you more."

"But you said all premiums are the same."

"Yes, but all plans have a yearly cost plus your monthly premiums."

You're confused. "That doesn't make any sense. Isn't it semantics? Wouldn't you simply take the yearly total and add that to twelve months of premiums, and that's your total cost?"

"I wouldn't try to understand it," she says, becoming visibly irritated.

You press onward. "What would I get for the Bronze plan as opposed to the Platinum plan?"

"Well, the Bronze plan has fewer services that are included."

"But the president said that all insurance companies are required to offer the same mandates."

"Well," she says, "not exactly. There's a basic level of mandates or benefits that are offered, but then there are additional benefits that aren't offered."

"Like what?"

"Take this Bronze plan. For women without a personal history of breast cancer, the federal government says that they need a mammogram starting at age fifty and then every other year after that."

You say, "But, the American Cancer Society suggests your first mammogram at age forty followed by every other year until age fifty, then yearly after age fifty."[10]

The women responds, "With the Bronze and Silver plans, we follow the government guidelines suggesting a women's first mammogram should be performed at age fifty, but with the Gold and Platinum plans, we follow the American Cancer Society recommendations."

This example is just one possibility of what these insurance exchanges will include. The specifics of which plans will be offered and how they will be offered is up to the states as long as they comply with the mandates as set forth by the PPACA and by the HHS secretary. If the states fail to comply, or if some of the plans do not include every specific mandate, then the federal government will step in and provide their own plans from which the uninsured people can choose.

Also, I would be remiss if I didn't point out one of the important misrepresentations made frequently by the PPACA supporter crowd. The PPACA supporters want Americans to believe and accept that there currently are no reasonable methods for our citizens to find affordable health insurance policies. This is disingenuous, as the free market has presented America with many reasonable and affordable health insurance solutions in the last decade or even longer. If I am shopping for an affordable policy that meets the specific medical needs of me and my family, I can look no further than to the health insurance broker. The independent broker is the consumer advocate, with regards to identifying each individuals and each families health insurance needs, and then the broker does just that. They communicate directly with the large health insurance companies, and broker a unique plan that specifically provides the current health insurance needs for the individual or the family.

As is generally the case, when the government gets out of the way and allows the free market to present our citizens with their solutions, the competition does one of several things, it assures quality, promotes accessibility, and demands affordability. That's how Capitalism or supply side economics works, regardless of the goods and services being provided... even in the health insurance industry.

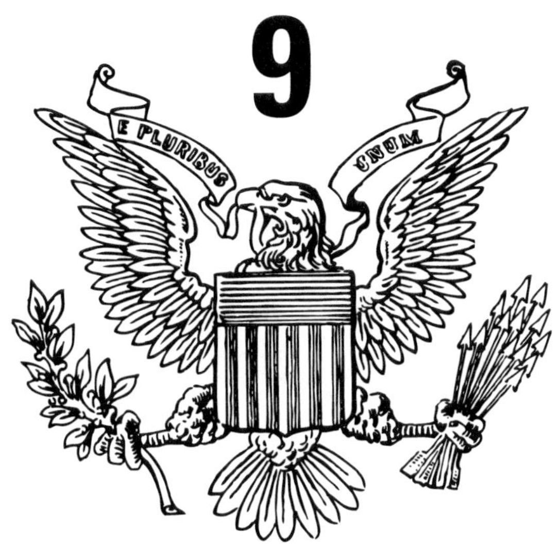

9

PHYSICIAN SHORTAGE

One of the most important issues facing the American health care industry is a physician shortage crisis. As a country, we throw around the word "crisis" liberally. Just because we face a societal problem doesn't mean we have a crisis on our hands. Is the shortage of doctors in our country really of crisis proportion? When you see the numbers, you, too, may be convinced "crisis" is an accurate description.

CURRENT NUMBERS

This could be an even larger problem than you may realize. According to the Association of American Medical Colleges (AAMC), in 2010, 954,000 doctors in the United States had active medical licenses. A physician can have an active license and yet be retired, so this number is slightly inflated because there are at least

30,000 doctors with active licenses who are not currently practicing their trade. Of these 954,000 doctors, 352,908 were PCPs.[1]

Did you know that there already is a significant shortage of PCPs? The problem is ominous, depending on which source you choose to refer to. The American College of Physicians (ACP) reported in a 2009 peer-reviewed study an estimated shortage of 35,000 to 44,000 PCPs for adults by 2025[2]. The AAMC says the country could face a shortage of as many as 150,000 doctors by the same year and that, once the PPACA health reform bill is fully implemented, about 45,000 more PCPs will be necessary by 2020 to meet the growing number of patients having health insurance and finally seeking the care they have neglected. The AAMC also projects a shortage of 33,100 doctors in cardiology, oncology, and emergency medicine.[3]

Health care reform is not a new idea, and the shrinking number of physicians in America didn't happen overnight. Therefore, it is logical that this problem was identified long ago and that forward thinking and proactive planning were obviously enacted before a real crisis could actually develop, correct? Well, perhaps not exactly.

PCPs provide more than 50 percent of all ambulatory care visits, 80 percent of patient visits for hypertension, and 69 percent of visits for both chronic obstructive pulmonary disease and diabetes.[4] Yet, they comprise only one-third of the US doctor workforce, according to the ACP. If the current trend continues, fewer than one in five physicians will be in an adult primary care specialty.

The Council on Graduate Medical Education has recommended that compensation to PCPs be increased to 70 percent of the average payment for physician specialties to train and retain a sufficient supply of PCPs.[5]

Following these recommendations, and with our attention directly placed on health care reform and Congress's desire to directly face all these real problems, like a shortage of PCP's, Congress has implemented changes, right? The PPACA recognizes this potential PCP shortage and proposes a 10 percent boost in current Medicare payments to PCPs.[6] Too little, too late!

MEDICAL EDUCATION

Of course, Congress must have adequately addressed the education side, creating attractive incentives and education opportunities that encourage medical students to enter into primary care, yes?

In 2009, about 18,000 students entered US medical schools.[7] In 2010, after the PPACA passed Congress, four new medical schools opened with a total enrollment of 190 students, and another twelve medical schools increased their enrollment by another 150 students for a total of 340 additional medical students—not an overwhelming influx that would solve the PCP shortage. Now, we know that doctors had to have seen 25 percent more patients in 2010 than they did in 1990 to maintain an equivalent income,[8] and with the influx of patients with the PPACA we can simply expect these PCPs to see twice as many patients. For their efforts, they will receive a whopping 10 percent increase in their Medicare fees!

There is also a shortage of medical resident positions. Residency is the period of postgraduate education when medical graduates receive their specialty training. In the 1970s and early 1980s, a medical school graduate had the choice of completing an internship and then entering general practice, or the graduate could enter a residency in the area of specialization that he or she chose. In the mid to late 1980s, fewer medical graduates completed an internship. Instead, all areas of medicine provided residency training in their specific specialty. In addition, the area of general medicine developed its own specialty, known as family medicine. So, if your doctor is truly a general practitioner (GP), he probably completed only an internship rather than a three-year residency in family medicine. He may have been allowed to not complete the residency of family medicine because of a grandfather clause but sit for the boards in family medicine and then be able to declare himself a board-certified GP. But after 1990, essentially anyone in America who entered general medicine actually completed a three-year residency in family medicine and thus became an FP, which is the specialty residency training for the general medicine specialist. Therefore, the specialty of general practice is family medicine.

To specifically address the PCP shortage in America, Congress must have studied the current medical education trends and developed a reasonable solution for this problem, correct? There are 110,000 resident positions in this country, according to the AAMC.[9] Residencies at teaching hospitals rely on Medicare funding for each resident slot. Currently, there is a shortage of resident positions in America. In other words, there is not a resident slot in all areas of primary care and all specialties for each medical school graduate. Because teaching hospitals rely heavily on Medicare funding to pay for each of their residency slots,[10] it would make sense that Congress would recognize the residency position shortage and act accordingly. Here's what they did: In 1997, Congress placed a cap on funding for medical residencies. Teaching hospitals stated unequivocally that this cap hurt their ability to expand the number of resident positions. Doctors' groups and hospitals expected that Congress would hear their pleas to lift this cap and increase Medicare funding in the new health reform legislation. To the chagrin of the hospitals and the doctors (and, for that matter, the country), a provision to raise the cap or increase the residency funding was NOT included in the PPACA. Yes, once again, when Congress had the opportunity to provide a real solution to a serious problem—a crisis—they turned their heads and looked the other way, something to which we have all grown accustomed!

MID-LEVELS

But Congress did not completely ignore the primary care shortage; they did focus some of their attention on NPs and PAs for filling our PCP positions around the country. NPs make up one of the fastest growing professions in this country, with 140,000 NPs qualified to practice in America in 2010.[11] This is a significant two-year increase from 125,000 in 2008, and it's quite a difference from the increase in 340 medical school graduates from 2009 to 2010.

Did you know that NPs and registered nurses with master's degrees and, in some cases, PhDs are trained to perform many of the same tasks as your FP? Family NPs need four years for a Bachelor of Science in Nursing, two years for a Master of Nursing or three or four years for a PhD of Nursing (depending on the program), and in some cases one year of postgraduate family medicine training (similar to residency training but only one year instead of three years) for a total of either seven, eight, or nine years of education, depending on the program. FPs need four years for an Undergraduate Bachelor of Science, four years of medical school, and three years of family medicine residency for a total of eleven years of education.[12]

NPs cost the health care system less money for education, fewer years to completion of a degree, and lower salaries than their counterpart FPs. Of course, Congress is trying to make our health system less costly, and they see NPs assisting in this manner. It's only a matter of time before your PCP on your new health plan is an NP.

Then there's the PA. The same logic holds true regarding overall cost to the system. PA educational training requires four years for an Undergraduate Bachelor of Science and four years of PA graduate school for a total of eight years of education. Again, it's easy to see why these two professions are so attractive to the health reform program and how they will fulfill an important role while providing a logical solution to the primary care shortage crisis.

DOCTORS OR PROVIDERS?

In fact, to the doctor's chagrin, the new and politically correct moniker for anyone who delivers health care in America is now "provider". Although this change is subtle and might appear insignificant, it is anything but that. This intentional change of title has the purpose of appearing non-judgmental. In our world of tolerance, the new label is all inclusive. Anyone who engages in the delivery of health care is no longer to be identified by the level of their training or their qualifications, but instead is to be lumped into a catch-all category of "provider". When a clinician is singled out based on their level of education, there is a chance that someone might be offended or might feel their medical training is inferior to the doctor. Never mind that there is a distinct and measurable difference in the various levels of education.

Next time you are in a hospital, see if the health care workers refer to those people who are administering medical treatment to patients as "doctors" or as "providers". I suspect you may be surprised at what you hear. As a doctor, who spent four years in undergraduate education, four years in medical school, three years in family medicine residency, four years in diagnostic radiology residency, and one year in interventional radiology fellowship post-graduate medical education, I strongly believe that I have earned the right to distinguish myself from the other clinical providers (NP's and PA's) by a meaningful title of doctor. I do not feel that I should need to apologize, or water down the differences between my education and that of other medical providers. Unfortunately, the label discussion has been framed by individuals who are not even in the business of practicing medicine, but rather are in the business of promoting class warfare, dividing groups of American's, and diluting traditional standards and qualifications. It wasn't that long ago the people who entered into a doctor's examination room included the doctor, his patient, and perhaps a nurse or assistant. Now, besides these players, members of CMS, representatives from HHS, officials from Congress, and politically correct advocates have inappropriately forced themselves into the doctor's examination room, too.

ATTRITION

Besides having a physician shortage, there is the current exodus of physicians leaving the workforce. I read about a physician from Arizona who declared in April 2010 that he would be leaving his practice and heading into early retirement. He received significant attention for his actions, and he was interviewed by Neil Cavuto on Fox News.[13] The physician was frustrated and left the medical practice because he could no longer sustain, or stomach, the continual accusations placed on physicians by Medicare. He cited the recent increase in the amount of the potential monetary fine as defined by 2011 changes to Medicare regulations for fraud and abuse by doctors who participate in Medicare. In the past, the fine for Medicare "fraud" per infraction was $10,000. That in itself was exorbitant. Recently, the CMS and HHS raised this fine to $50,000 per infraction.[14]

MEDICARE ABUSE

This physician's specific concerns about Medicare received some scrutiny from uninformed bloggers, questioning that he must be hiding something if he allowed the possibility of a $50,000 fine to scare him out of medicine. What is a real crying shame is this is often the impression of a misinformed public. In fact, President Obama and his administration have frequently and boldly stated there is overwhelming fraud and abuse in Medicare and that policing the providers of Medicare, catching these abusers, and fining them was how we would be able to pay for a significant portion of the expenses associated with the PPACA. If the public continually hears this from the White House and from the media, of course they would begin to believe that this statement must be true.

Let's take a closer look at the so-called abuse of Medicare. A patient's doctor orders a CT scan of the head. The Medicare patient takes the handwritten order to the hospital and proceeds to schedule a CT scan of the head without contrast. The radiology technician questions the patient and finds that, besides suffering from recent headaches, he also has had a seizure. The tech then asks the radiologist (the physician specialist for radiology) if the patient should have the CT with or without IV contrast. The test of choice for new-onset seizures is with IV contrast, so the radiologist says (acting as an appropriate consultant and specialist) to do the CT with IV contrast. Medicare will pay about $15 more for the CT study of the head with IV contrast than without IV contrast. Here's the catch: It seems absolutely appropriate that the radiologist, who is the expert regarding diagnostic imaging studies, has the right and the authority to change the PCP's order to a CT with IV contrast. In fact, if the radiologist and his staff are astute enough to catch this incorrect or less-beneficial order, they should be rewarded as the CMS champion who is trying to do the right test for the best chance of making an accurate diagnosis and also the most cost-effective practice of radiology. If he didn't catch this incorrect order and the patient had the CT without IV contrast, the radiologist would interpret the study, see that the patient had a history of a new-onset seizure, and recommend that the patient have a second CT with IV contrast. Not discovering and correcting this order would ultimately lead to more than double the expenses to the CMS rather than simply a $15 increase for the best test from the get-go.

Who, if anyone, gets in trouble with the CMS in this example? Who do you think should? Well, because the CMS is a government agency made up of thousands of regulations and rules, under the strictest rules of Medicare the radiologist has just committed "fraud" by changing the PCP's order and, if "caught," would be fined for his "fraudulent" behavior. But that's not all. The radiologist actually broke two rules: He changed a doctor's order, and he billed for the CT study of the head with contrast, which was an "illegally" ordered study. The radiologist's intention in this case was to do the right thing for the patient, the system, and the American taxpayers who are paying all the bills; however, in the eyes of the CMS and our government, he has broken the law and is now a common criminal.

Another extremely common example is a visit to the doctor's office. To standardize payment, the CMS established a coding system with five different levels of office visits: 99211, 99212, 99213, 99214, and 99215.[15] Each of these codes has a specific list of criteria that must be met for appropriate reimbursement. For example, a patient sees the doctor for a short office visit because of an earache. The doctor proceeds to examine the patient. On the basis of the amount of time, the different systems examined (ear-nose-throat being one system and the chest being a second system), and the difficulty of the medical diagnosis and treatment, the doctor looks at the specific criteria for each level of office visit and determines which number to assign. The lowest, most basic, and simplest office visit is 99211. In this example, the level of visit is probably a 99212, in which a short amount of time was spent with the patient, two systems were evaluated, and the diagnosis and treatment were straightforward. Unfortunately, the coding for office visits has been a huge source for claiming fraud and abuse by the CMS "police." This system of assigning the level of acuity with each particular office visit is not in any way straightforward. It's extremely difficult to make medicine and the practice-of-medicine cookbook.

Here's the real rub: The doctor has a thirty-forty-minute visit with Mrs. Smith, his favorite octogenarian. He does a thorough physical exam. Mrs. Smith always has a "grocery list" of medical problems she wishes to address, many of which are the same items she discusses every quarterly visit. The doctor fills out her seven scripts, proving a high complexity of acuity. However, because the doctor is a fair and decent guy, he decides to code Mrs. Smith's office visit as a 99213, even though he knows he could probably justify a 99214 or even a 99215. But he realizes many of these issues are always the same, he now knows Mrs. Smith's medical problems as if they were his own, and he feels it is wrong to soak the system for the higher-level-of-acuity office visit.

Well, here's the problem: Medicare calls any fluctuation from the guidelines (yes, they are called guidelines, or recommendations; they are not etched in stone!) as failing to follow the rules, and in the strictest sense this is fraud and abuse—never mind that the doctor just saved the system $40 or up to $80. This coding-down happens in every medical office many times over every single day. Once the CMS comes in, does an audit, and declares that this doctor (who frequently codes-down on office visits) has 250 infractions over the last month, how on earth would this doctor ever pay the potential $50,000 fine for each infraction! Then there are the severe and detrimental effects that this news will have on the doctor's reputation once the general public and his patients hear that he's engaging in Medicare fraud and had 250 infractions to boot. Do you suppose the public will understand that these are ridiculous variations from the rules to begin with and that the doctor should actually be praised for his frugal and practical behavior and the manner in which he saved the Medicare system significant money? I don't think so. I suspect the patients and the public will look at the now-criminalized doctor with disdain and disgust! These are some of the real and practical problems doctors face every single day in America, and it's these types of issues that have sent physicians running from their profession into early retirement. Do you blame them?

SHORTAGE OF PCP'S

Three in ten doctors become FPs. The number of medical students specializing in primary care has decreased by more than 50 percent since the late 1990s.[16] As baby boomers age and the number of seniors increases over the next decade, there will be an even greater demand for PCPs. The AAFP predicted in 2009 there would be a shortage of 40,000 family doctors over the next ten years.[17] In 2009, a Merritt Hawkins survey of PCPs revealed that 10 percent of doctors who responded were planning on leaving medicine within the next three years.[18] Also in 2009, *Investor's Business Daily* conducted a poll that revealed 45 percent of doctors would consider early retirement if the PPACA passed, and of course we know it did. The same survey also revealed that 67 percent of practicing physicians believed that fewer students would apply for medical school over the next decade if the PPACA passed.[19]

To gain a plausible understanding of physician practice and decision trends, we can look closely at Massachusetts, where state health care reform was enacted in 2006 and serves as a model for health care trends. Massachusetts citizens saw an increase of 440,000 patients to the ranks of the insured. These former uninsured patients were added to state Medicaid and government-funded health insurance plans. What Massachusetts found was an instant worsening of its previous physician shortage within the state. Many Massachusetts doctors have retired, moved out of state, or quit the practice of medicine. One well-documented statement came from an Amherst FP who told the New York Times in 2008 that eighteen of her colleagues had already left Massachusetts. Patient waiting lists apparently increased to record levels, with 1,500 patients at some clinics.[20]

Generally, when there is a shortage of doctors but the demand for medical care increases, like the current situation America is facing, either the price for medical treatment goes up because of supply and demand or the government steps in and controls prices while dictating who receives what medical care. Isn't this rationing of health care, something that we were promised would not be permitted to happen to our health care system under the health reform plan? This is exactly what Massachusetts has observed. Health care costs in the Bay State have increased at an even faster rate than the national average, and the state government has stepped in and implemented a system of capitation in which health care providers receive a fixed fee for each patient they care for.

ELECTRONIC MEDICAL RECORDS

Another reason for this premature departure of doctors, retiring earlier than they initially would have predicted, is the additional financial strains placed on already overextended practices. For example, in 2008, Congress passed the electronic health records (EHRs) stimulus package. This legislation recommended that nonhospital-based physicians purchase EHR programs and software for their office practices. For financial incentive, the program stated that doctors must purchase and implement a qualified and fully functioning EHR program for meaningful use by 2011 or face decreasing Medicare payments. Government subsidies were earmarked and available to doctors who complied with this suggestion. However, if doctors failed to comply by 2015, they would see a 1 percent decrease in their Medicare payments; if they failed to comply by 2016, they would see a 2 percent decrease; if they failed to comply by 2017, they would see a 3 percent decrease; and so on for each following year.[21] Even though participation in the implementation of the EHR program was elective, the government placed some strong incentives to participate in this laborious and expensive process. (I would not refer to a decrease in fee schedule as an incentive but rather a fine or punishment.)

What exactly is the purpose of the EHR? The benefits are supposed to be numerous. In theory, this electronic record would eliminate paper, improve throughput, improve efficiency, eventually decrease overall expenses and overhead, and enable instant access and portability. The idea was also to provide clinical tools to determine patient treatment outcomes. For example, if a patient were marked as having diabetes, the EHR would alert the provider that a hemoglobin A1C test (a long-term diabetes-control laboratory test) was needed.

But like many of the suggested government programs, it's been wrought with difficulties and concerns. The systems have proved expensive, costing anywhere from $50,000 to $250,000 to implement, based on the level of functions offered and the number of providers using the system. The requirements of the legislation become more stringent with each passing year. Meaningful-use criteria (or in other words, implementations of EHR's) must be met by 2011. Certification of qualified EHRs must be completed by 2013. More stringent requirements are planned for 2015, like appropriate but mandatory software updates. Then there are the patient practice requirements such as maintaining up-to-date medication and allergy lists on all patients in the database, having the physician or his staff electronically prescribe (Script Pad, Inc.) at least 75 percent of the time, and incorporating at least 50 percent of the laboratory studies into the EHR, all by the end of 2011. If these criteria are not met, the physician is not in compliance and risks a fine or decrease in Medicare payments.

This type of patient medical-management electronic tool has a couple of great benefits, with one of the greatest being the e-prescribing capabilities. Unfortunately, most of the 130 vendors of the so-called qualified EHRs failed to allot the necessary time and attention in developing a sophisticated e-prescribing tool that truly assists doctors and their patients. However, there is a company, Script Pad, Inc. that has performed exhaustive and effective research and has taken the time to fully understand the prescription-writing needs and demands of a busy physician.[22] Script Pad's particular e-prescribing tool can be fully integrated into each of the qualified EHR plans. In my experience, the current e-prescribing tools of nearly every one of the EHR programs are poor to average at best. The minimal extra cost to gain excellent functionality and to provide improved efficiency as well as increased patient and physician satisfaction is absolutely worth it. Even though I am not a big supporter of the recommended implementation of EHRs in all physician practices, I am completely sold on the superior functionality of Script Pad's prescription software. If physicians choose to take the Medicare pay cuts and not implement a qualified EHR, I'd still recommend they at least implement this Script Pad's software to their practice. This program is highly sophisticated: It recalls past prescriptions; communicates with the pharmacies electronically; and, most importantly, identifies and alerts the physician of the medications on each individual insurance plan's formulary to maximize patient satisfaction and results and minimize patient cost and time spent waiting at the pharmacy for a prescription to be filled. All physicians who want to enhance their current practice should strongly consider Script Pad for their electronic prescription needs!

Turning our attention back to the problems associated with the EHRs, doctors are concerned that this is one step closer to our government completely taking over our health care system. It gives the government way too much access to all our information. And when an EHR is fully integrated with the PPACA, Uncle Sam will always be watching over your and your doctor's shoulders. This causes significant anxiety. Will the government begin to tell doctors that the treatment they prescribed is not the acceptable treatment, and therefore the government will not pay for the service?

NEW COMMITTEES

Of the many new committees or boards included in the PPACA, the Patient-Centered Outcomes Research Institute (PCORI) is a nineteen-member research board of directors[23] (imagine the salaries of these federal employees!) appointed by the secretary of the HHS. Their responsibility is to study each of the various acceptable treatments for each particular disease state to determine the expected best outcome. Say you were to contract walking pneumonia, generally caused by a bacterium called *Mycoplasma pneumoniae.* Your doctor prescribes Ciprofloxin because you had a similar lung infection last year and responded to that treatment. But the PCORI has already studied the many different treatment options for walking pneumonia, and they have determined that the best and most cost-effective treatment is penicillin. They deny payment for your medication, even though you will respond effectively to this drug. That's one of the problems with governments getting involved in medicine; they tend to take away the doctor's ability to practice medicine based on his experiences and knowledge of his patients' medical histories and their relationships. Medicine becomes a one-size-fits-all practice. Oh, sure, Cipro isn't that costly these days, so you can afford to pay for this out of your own pocket, if you like. But what if the disease were a rare form of, say, an adenoid adenocarcinoma of the sinus, and the medication that the government will pay for is the cheaper but less-effective chemotherapy? Yet, you had responded to the more-expensive chemotherapeutic regimen only three years ago. Now that you are suffering from a recurrence of the same cancer, you want the same effective and proven treatment; however, it costs tens of thousands of dollars. What do you do? To pay for this out of your pocket may not be practical or even possible, so are you forced to accept the PCORI-recommended outcomes-based treatment? You can see the many problems government intervention can cause.

According to the Federal Trade Commission, another problem facing Americans is medical identity theft. Could identity thieves be using your personal and health insurance information to get medical treatment, prescription drugs, or surgery?[24] Picture this: You receive a bill from your insurance company that says you still owe $8,400 for your sexual reassignment surgery. An enclosed letter from your doctor states, "Dear Ms. Smith, I hope you are recovering well from your recent transgender surgery. I know this can be a difficult surgery both physically and emotionally. Because of the numerous additional medications and ancillary medical services you will probably need during this transitional period of your life, and because this is not my area of expertise in family medicine, I will no longer be able to provide you medical care. I took the liberty to refer your information onto Dr. Jones, as this is one of his areas of interest and expertise. His office will be contacting you in the near future. Best of luck. Your Doctor. Dr. Joe Public"

Now, think of the repercussions, even though HIPAA laws strictly state that your medical information is to remain confidential. Imagine the horror when you think of your friends and friend of a friend who work at the insurance company, your doctor's office, and Dr. Jones's office, not to mention the problems you now face with repairing your medical and financial identities. In fact, simply pondering medical identity theft and the many problems this could cause you and your family is sobering. But this couldn't happen with the strict oversight placed on your doctor and your insurance company to keep your personal medical and health insurance information confidential, right? People may feel secure with their general information, that is, until they look at the amount of identity theft in America and hear the horror stories about everyday citizens whose identities were stolen and how difficult it has been for them to repair the damage and restore their lives. With a qualified EHR, all your medical and health insurance information is right there, in one little file stored on the new office computer system, at any identity thief's fingertips.

If, by chance, your doctor has recently committed to purchasing the recommended EHR program, an extremely important question for him or his office personnel is, "What safety measures have been taken to secure my health information?" You may want to even go so far as to ask if he has included LifeLock with his new EHR program. LifeLock has become the national leader regarding protecting identities.[25] Their sophisticated methods to secure and protect your information are amazing. Having turned to LifeLock, I'm now convinced breaking into Fort Knox would be easier than breaking into my LifeLock-secured personal information. (Of course, I hear the government has spent all the gold, and there's simply a small note on a chair that says "IOU three tons of gold, Uncle Sam.")

So, it's a culmination of each of these issues and more that has sent many doctors running toward retirement as fast as they can. Do you blame them? Not to worry; we have 340 more medical school applicants and thousands of more NPs and PAs coming to the rescue. To quote the titular character in the movie *Mrs. Doubtfire*, as she leaps over the short wall at the restaurant to administer the Heimlich maneuver to Pierce Brosnan's character, "Help is on the way, dear!" And it takes the form of our government!

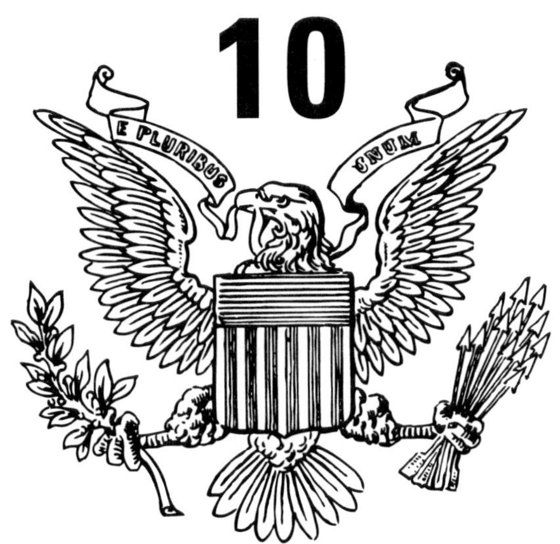

10

IS OUR CURRENT SYSTEM REALLY THAT BAD?

Our current health delivery system and our level of medical care and expertise have taken a large beating by the media and Congress, especially since we began the debate on health care reform in early 2008, which ultimately lead to the passage of the PPACA in March 2010. Was all this criticism legitimate, or were the facts twisted and distorted for an even greater agenda? I'll let you be the judge.

There have been plenty of reasons to complain about the rapidly increasing costs of health care plans and insurance premiums in America over the past decade. The increase in costs has been exponential. I have also frequently heard that the American health system is actually one of the less-effective systems in the world,[1] and I've often wondered how this could even begin to be true.

I've been in medicine for twenty-five years. I've completed two residencies and a fellowship. I've observed some of the most amazing technological advances in American health care in only two and a half decades. To say that our system of medical care is second to any other country is mind boggling. I've frequently heard that our average life expectancy, as a nation, ranks lower than that of most powerful countries around the globe.[2] I've read that our infant mortality rate is poor, at best, when compared with that of other countries.[3] And, of course, I've observed that the overall expense of our health care system is much higher than the rest of the world's.

Well, then, let's just take a close, critical, and analytical look at these allegations to see exactly how our current health system measures up to the rest of the world. According to the World Health Organization (WHO), life expectancy in America in 2009 was forty-second in the world, which was below most developed nations and some developing nations. In 2000, the WHO ranked the US health system as the highest in cost, first in responsiveness, thirty-seventh in overall performance, and seventy-second in overall health (among 191 member nations included in the study).[4]

As a doctor, I've had the privilege of delivering babies into this world and being at many patients' bedside as they passed on. I've watched the age of our geriatric population increase during my twenty-five years in medicine. The very first patient whose hospital care I participated in was an eighty-four-year-old man who had been bedridden for the six months before hospitalization. When he had a cardiac arrest, I was the first responder who began his advanced life support, administering cardiopulmonary resuscitation (CPR). I pulled the cord over his bed to announce a code blue, and within sixty seconds this debilitated, elderly man received instant heroic treatment in an attempt to restart his heart. The efforts were futile, however, and he died. The cost to the Medicare system back in 1989 was well over $30,000.

In my career alone, I've observed firsthand the high quality of the medical care delivered to Americans. Yes the costs are expensive but most things of significant value come at a price.

I've witnessed unbelievable advances in medical treatment from all areas of health care, such as improved medications, more-sophisticated surgical techniques, and highly technical diagnostic capabilities. After we have a patient swallow a microscopic camera, we can take a video of the inside of this patient's gastrointestinal (GI) system. Over the spring of 2011, recent advances to this tiny camera were announced to the nation. It now has mechanical fins that can be operated from a computerized joystick, allowing it to swim around in your GI system to take a closer look at any area of concern inside your stomach or intestines.[5]

In 2000, my father-in-law died of an aortic aneurysm rupture. He was a few months shy of eighty-two. I can't say for certain that he would still be alive today, but since his death the amazing technical advances in the treatment of thoracic and abdominal aortic aneurysms have progressed to amazing heights. I'm convinced he would have lived for at least several more years, and I doubt he would have died of his aneurysm. We can now insert a large stent through the artery in the leg and use x-ray guidance to place the stent (or a covered patch) inside the aorta to prevent an aneurysm from expanding and ultimately popping.

My own mother would not be alive today had it not been for the rapid response of the emergency personnel and the technological advances of the automatic electric defibrillator (AED), which is now available in most community buildings in this country. I lived only two miles from my mother when she had her heart attack, so I was the first responder. She coded in front of me and I began CPR. My father met the firemen at the curb and alerted them to bring in the AED. Within two minutes, my mother's heart was electrically restarted, and, because of significant technological advances, she's alive and well today.

CURRENT RANKING

I've observed these and hundreds of other amazing advances in our medical care right here in America. Most of these advances come from our American scientific community and from the research-and-development divisions of our private sector pharmaceutical and medical device companies. So, when I read these statistics or hear that our health system is second to any other country, I am skeptical. But the numbers don't lie…or do they?

Because it has been difficult for me to believe that our life expectancy rate of 78.7 years is poorer than that of other countries, I decided to research how these statistics are collected. Did you know in 2007America has the highest motor vehicle accident (MVA) rate per capita (14.4 deaths/100,000) compared with all the other countries? I suspect this is because of our wealth and that nearly every household has at least two cars. Unfortunately, all these motor vehicles have translated to an increased mortality rate. Did you know that America has one of the highest homicide rates compared with other United Nations countries?[6] Why does this matter? The homicide rate includes the overall deaths of Americans who are younger than our oldest citizens; therefore, when you include each of these homicides in our life expectancy rate, you can see how the murders of these citizens have decreased the average age at which our citizens die. This gives a misleading appearance to our overall average life expectancy. In fact, if you subtract the statistics of the Americans who die prematurely in MVAs and from homicide, our average life expectancy goes well over eighty years. When compared with other United Nations countries, four countries are tied for eighth on the WHO life expectancy list: Israel, Macau, France, and Canada at 80.7 years.[7] Our newly calculated life expectancy would place us at or above these four countries, which is a significant difference from being ranked forty-second.

The United Nations World Population Prospects report from April 2009 ranked America thirty-fourth in infant mortality among the list of the 197 United Nations member countries included in the report. Infant mortality is measured as the number of infant deaths per 1,000 live births. The average infant mortality rate was 42.09 for the 197 United Nations countries and 49.4 for the world as a whole. America's average infant mortality rate was 7.07 in 2009, which is an improvement from 30.46 in 1950.[8]

This overall infant mortality rate does not paint a flattering portrait of our health care system. In fact, shouldn't much of our greatest attention as physicians be focused on the infants and newborns in our country? Taking into consideration these figures, having your baby in America looks pretty glum. With these statistics, wouldn't the illegal immigrants want to return to their own homelands to improve their newborn infants' chances of survival? But that is not what I've observed with our health care system. In fact, when I was a resident in family medicine at one of the tertiary care teaching hospitals that administer indigent care to the poorer citizens of Kansas City, I treated several brand new American citizens in the neonatal unit. Their young illegal immigrant mothers had not received prenatal care for fear of being deported back to their homelands and had arrived at the emergency department in premature labor. It amazed us young doctors in training just how precise the young women's timing had to be to feel confident that they would indeed progress to precipitous labor and definitely deliver (even if the newborn were preterm). If their timing were to prove too soon, the emergency personnel would have to quickly administer tocolytic medication in an attempt to halt their labor and delivery, at which point their alien status would be discovered and they would be deported to their native countries. In fact, I never saw a preterm labor effectively halted during my residency training, but I participated in myriad deliveries of new American citizens.

Recalling my own experiences, I observed sophisticated and compassionate neonatal medical care throughout my training and during my years of medical practice. So, how could these numbers claim that we have such a poor infant mortality rate? I dived right into the middle of this issue expecting to find that we somehow neglected our poor, even though my experiences suggested just the opposite regarding medical care. Here's what I found out: We do take good care of our poor. We provide high-level and consistent prenatal and perinatal medical care to these women in our society. The young mothers on Medicare do receive quality obstetric medical care.

Then why is there a high infant mortality rate in our country? Is it because for every thousand deliveries, no matter how good the care, a few of these newborns will die no matter what? This proved true. However, if this offered the correct explanation, then wouldn't every country's infant mortality rate be the same unless a country actually tried to neglect its pregnant citizens? What country would do that? Certainly not America.

The answer to this riddle may surprise you. If you worked for the WHO and your assignment was to study and determine the infant mortality of the United Nations countries of the world, wouldn't you use the same standard or same definitions for your research to be certain of standardization? Isn't that the main purpose of any research or collection of data, to be certain that you are comparing apples to apples and not apples to oranges? Well, there's a great controversy about what constitutes infant mortality. Is that hard to believe? It isn't if you understand why. Think of it like this: At what point is a fetus a viable infant? When is the newborn considered survivable or capable of living on its own? Does the fetus become viable or will the newborn survive if and when it reaches twenty-three weeks, thirty weeks, or thirty-four weeks? This same discrepancy exists regarding prolife and prochoice discussions. The prochoice crowd likes to refer to an unborn baby as a nonviable tissue mass. (If I am prolife, does that mean I'm antichoice, based on the converse?) Thirty years ago in America, the earliest gestation age for survival was about thirty weeks. Now, the gestation age of survivability in America has decreased to about twenty-three weeks.[9]

Every country determines its own definition of infant survivability and, in turn, infant mortality. For example, in Switzerland, an infant must be thirty centimeters in length at birth before it is considered a living baby. Therefore, if a premature infant is born and dies but measures less than thirty centimeters, the birth is not included in the mortality rate. In France and Belgium, a newborn must be at least twenty-six weeks of gestation age to be counted in the statistics; newborns at twenty-five weeks of gestation age who die at birth are not included in the infant mortality numbers. If they aren't even included, then they can't be considered a negative statistic.

What about America? We have one of (if not the most) sophisticated neonatology medical systems in the world. In fact, if high-risk pregnancies can be transferred, both Canada and Mexico go through significant efforts to transfer these high-risk infants to America before delivery, as the infants will have the greatest chance of survival. If these high-risk infants die, they are included in America's infant mortality rate, not Canada's or Mexico's! In August 2007, the *Calgary Herald* from Calgary, Canada, reported that a pregnant Calgarian woman with identical quadruplets delivered in a Montana hospital. The woman was transferred to Benefis Hospital in Montana when she began showing signs of going into labor because no Canadian hospital had enough neonatal intensive-care beds for all four babies.[10]

In America, we follow the strict WHO suggestions, which state that if an infant shows any signs of life, it is considered a live birth,[11] regardless of gestation age or length. Therefore, any infant who is delivered and shows any signs of life is included in the infant mortality rate, whether the mother's preterm labor began at nineteen weeks and the infant was delivered and died or if the high-risk set of quadruplets from Calgary were brought to America and they were delivered and then died. If children are stillborn and are past the age of viability (currently, somewhere around twenty-two weeks of gestation age), they are included in America's infant mortality statistics. Any infants born on American soil are included in the statistics. Frankly, I'm surprised we don't include our abortions when calculating our infant mortality rate.

You can see that we are rigid regarding our infant mortality statistics, certainly much more strict than most other countries. One of the more intriguing twists to recording infant mortality is that the more sophisticated our neonatology medical care becomes, and the earlier we enable a premature infant to survive (lowering the gestation age where we can enable survival), the higher the risk of infant mortality. Thus, if we continue to lower the gestation age of viability, we may see a greater number of infant mortalities. How's that for a negative distortion of our amazing technological advances?

It's actually insulting that America has had to listen to the diatribe and the innuendo that we somehow allowed and willingly accepted our forty-second-place ranking among other United Nations countries regarding infant mortality. To imply that we neglect our newborns when we compare our medical system and obstetric care with those of other countries is inaccurate and significantly misleading. Why are some of our own citizens more than willing to spout these statistics without attempting to gain a factual understanding of their country's wealthy, highly technical, and sophisticated medical system? The only explanation I can give is that they have an agenda that is greater than the actual facts and details to try to discredit America. It appears these people who gladly refer to this forty-second-place ranking in infant mortality want to imply that America is cold, heartless, and uncaring because we would ignore our most innocent and vulnerable national treasures, our unborn and newborn infants.[12]

In 2009, the US Census Bureau reported that a record 50.7 million American residents (16.7 percent) were uninsured. (It is interesting that they state "residents" in their report, for the number includes about 9.9 million illegal immigrants or, as they state, "noncitizens.") Also according the report, more money is spent on health care per person in America than in any other nation in the world. (If in no other category, we are number one!) A greater percentage of total income is spent on health care in America than in any United Nations member state except East Timor. The report states that although not all people are insured, America has the third-highest public health care expenditure per capita because of the high cost of medical care in the country.[13]

RISING COSTS

The Organization for Economic Co-operation and Development (OECD) reports that, since 1980, America has had one of the highest growth rates in per capita health care spending among higher-income countries. Health care spending around the world is generally rising at a faster rate than overall economic growth, so almost all countries have seen health care spending increase as a percentage of their gross domestic product (GDP) over time. In America, the share of GDP devoted to health care grew from 8.8 percent in 1980 to 15.2 percent in 2003 and to 16.3 percent in 2010. The Office of the Actuary (OACT) of the CMS estimated that America spent $2.26 trillion on health care or $7,439 per person in 2007, up from $2.1 trillion or $7,026 per person in 2006.[14]

By all accounts, it looks like health care in America is expensive. No matter how you look at the numbers, we unequivocally spend the most money on health care, including health insurance, when compared with all other countries. Have we always been this way?

There have been times in our nation's history when we stopped and pondered how something happened or why were all doing what we were doing. In 1942, Beardsley Ruml, one of the directors of the Federal Reserve Bank of New York, recommended to Congress the Current Tax Payment Act of 1943, in which employers assumed the responsibility of withholding federal income taxes from workers' paychecks and then directly paying the employees' taxes to the government on behalf of each worker. The act was signed into law by President Roosevelt.[15] Something as minor as this has caused more apathy about the amount of taxes being withheld than any other governmental decision in the past one hundred years. Whenever a significant responsibility or action is taken away from us, the natural tendency is to ignore the responsibility even exists. Since the turn of the century, there has been an awakening regarding our civic duty as citizens, albeit a slight awakening.

If you ask people how much money they make, most will tell you the amount of money they take home each pay period. Most people accurately know the amount of their paycheck, but if you rephrased the question and asked them how much money they pay toward state or federal income taxes or pay into the Federal Insurance Contributions Act (FICA) or Social Security and Medicare, a few of the more informed members of our society will know the percentages of their money that their employers hold and pay to the federal government on the employees' behalf (salaried employee: 6.2 percent Social Security and 1.45 percent Medicare, or 7.65 percent and the employer pays the other half).[16] But most employees could not begin to tell you exactly how much money is taken out of their checks each pay period to pay state, federal, and FICA taxes.

Had Beardsley Ruml left well enough alone and had not proposed his mandatory employer withholding program, I believe our taxes and our nation's debt would be much lower. If workers had instead received their paychecks at the end of each pay period and then had to write four checks payable to the federal government, the state government, the Social Security Administration, and the CMS, I believe the workers and taxpayers would have never let our taxes grow so high. When you have to write the check yourself, it changes your perspective. No longer would our society be apathetic toward how much money we each pay in taxes or to Social Security and Medicare. In this scenario, if Congress were to have the audacity to state that Medicare or Social Security were bankrupt, we would all be pretty darned upset because each us would know just how much we wrote our checks for every month.

Along this same line of thinking, this provides some of the insight into the expense of our health insurance. When we purchase goods or services, generally we buy them directly from the producer. If we buy groceries, we select our items and then pay for each one as we check out. We pay the plumber his going rate for his services. However, when we purchase health insurance, much of the time our employer writes the check to the insurance company on our behalf, much like the employer withholds our portion of state, federal, and FICA taxes. What this method of payment does is create employees who are apathetic about the cost of their health insurance. Whenever an employer or business assumes the responsibility for paying for a service, a couple of things happen over time: Whoever is providing the service often increases the price for it at a faster-than-reasonable rate, and whenever a business becomes the responsible party to make group decisions for the service, it often begins to look for ways to decrease the cost of that service. For example, when the service is health insurance, the insurance company often increases the cost of the health insurance or the premiums at an accelerated pace. The employer often looks for ways to find less-expensive insurance, or the employer who will not be able or willing to pay unlimited health benefits to its employees will begin to barter and bargain for health services, which ultimately leads to a form of rationed health care.

Of course, when your employer is paying for employees' health insurance, the employees are fine with allowing the boss to make those insurance decisions. The employees, over time, begin to lose touch with the rising cost of their health insurance. Before they realize it, the health insurance premiums have gone up considerably, but the number of paid-for benefits and services has dwindled. This leads to higher costs for less service, which has happened during the past two decades in America.

In 2007, $7,439 was spent on each person's health care in America. In 2009, 17.3 percent of America's GDP went to health care, the average American took $2,853 out of his or her pocket and used it on some form of medical care, and Americans spent $2,750 on eating out. According to the Bureau of Labor Statistics, in 2008, Americans spent 5.9 percent of their household budgets on health care, 12.8 percent on food, 17 percent on gasoline and transportation, and 33.9 percent on housing. It's true; we spend more on health care than do citizens of other countries, but we demand to receive better health care.[17]

CAN'T PUT A PRICE ON LIFE

I have heard family members say on countless occasions during the past twenty-four years that they wanted everything humanly possible for their family members' medical care to be performed. When faced with an ethical dilemma, such as a procedure that has a fairly high risk and expense but great reward, families have said, "Do everything you can to save dad's life." I recall a case where a seventy-two-year-old man had a sudden stroke. His speech was impaired, and half of his body was paralyzed. The diagnostic imaging showed a sudden clot in a major vessel in his brain. The heroic but most promising treatment for a near-complete to complete recovery was to slide a small catheter through the artery in his leg up through his body to his head. There, the catheter, using x-ray guidance, would be passed into the artery in the brain where the clot was blocking off blood flow. This highly technical, interventional, radiological procedure was expensive and risky but had a great chance for a significant recovery. I distinctly remember the conversation with the family; I told them the procedure was risky and that a couple of significantly bad things could happen. Their father could die from additional clots breaking loose and showering all the vessels in his brain, in turn cutting off the blood supply and the oxygen to his brain. Or, the extremely potent blood thinner that would be used to break up and dissolve the clot could cause their father to bleed from nearly anywhere in his body. The blood would become so thin that it could ultimately cause him to bleed internally. Or, the best outcome was that I could successfully place the catheter into the clot and dissolve it, reestablishing blood flow and oxygen to the brain. This would stop the stroke from progressing and lead to repair of the brain tissue. If I could accomplish this, their father would probably make a complete recovery. Two responses are seared in my brain. The wife broke down and could not regain her composure; the thought of her husband dying on the surgical table was more than she could bear. The daughter, observing all this, stated unwaveringly, "Money is no object; do whatever you can to save dad. If he dies in the process, he would rather die than be left in this state for the remainder of his life."

I've often wondered about those words "money is no object." This man had Medicare, and so the procedure would be covered. So, in essence, money was no object for the family. But what if they had been self-payers? Would money have then been an object? If money were the number-one concern and the family said, "Do everything you can until you reach $16,555. When you go above $16,556, stop. That is all we will be able to afford. Even if you're close to dissolving the clot, you'll have to stop." But what if the abbreviated treatment saved their father's life but left half of his body paralyzed? What then? Should I still stop? What about the postsurgical expenses like physical therapy? "Well, if you can go to

$16,555 and you've not accomplished dissolution of the clot, then you must be sure that dad dies, because he does not want to remain in this state. It's either all or none for this price."

Can you imagine such a conversation? I'm concerned that these types of rationing-of-care discussions may actually occur sometime soon. I hope this never happens while I'm practicing medicine. I've observed hundreds—perhaps thousands—of doctors as they have cared for patients. One of the most commonly heard statements from doctor to doctor, especially when the doctor is in a teaching role, is that our responsibility is to take care of patients, and if we maintain our focus and our attention on that goal and objective, then the money side or the insurance side will always work itself out. I, and most doctors I know, try to practice by this universal rule, and it has worked so far in my career for the past twenty-four years. I'm fearful that this rule may soon be obsolete.

We expect the best technology in America. If the best test is an MRI scan, then that's what each individual patient wants. If the surgery of choice is through a laparoscope, then no one wants an open procedure. If patients get cancer, their doctors want to give them the greatest chance for survival. If that means the newest medication or the most expensive chemotherapy, then that's what doctors want to provide for them in the form of treatment. Doctor's do NOT want to make decisions on medical treatment or medical care based on monetary influences.

Who among us can put a price tag on our health? If a young woman with three children at home develops breast cancer, and if there's a chance for a cure, then how much is that cure worth (1) to the patient, (2) to the patient's family, and (3) to society or to the expenses of the medical system? Breast cancer survival has improved steadily since 1990. That was not coincidental; Americans and pharmaceutical companies have spent millions of dollars to find a cure. In 2010, if a woman contracted stage 4 breast cancer that was previously known as incurable, she had a 20 percent chance (or one-in-five chance) of survival. How much is that worth? If the patient were you, how much is your life worth?

If the young woman in the above example tries the medication and is cured, how much is that cure worth? She owes her life to modern medicine. Doctors say that half of all medical treatments in use today were invented in the past twenty-five years, and much of this invention and research occurred right here in America. People come here from all over the world to receive their medical treatment. America leads the world in cancer treatment and survivability. In 1950, if you had a heart attack you had a 307-in-100,000 chance for survival. In 2000, you had a 126-in-100,000 chance of survival. The percentage of survival increased by more than 50 percent.[18] How much is that worth?

The survival rate among American women with breast cancer is 83.9 percent. In Great Britain, the survival rate is 69.7 percent. Patients with colon cancer have a 35 percent greater chance of survival if they receive their treatment in America as opposed to Great Britain. Men with prostate cancer in America have a 91.9 percent survival rate, but the survival rate is 73.7 percent in France and 51.1 percent in Great Britain. Where do you want to get your cancer therapy: Great Britain, France, or the good ol' USA?[19]

When you hear the next politician castigate the American health care system for the poor outcomes and the extreme costs, ask if this politician would like to go to another country—any other country—for medical care. None of these politicians speak of the amazing advances that have occurred in modern medicine because of the US commitment to technology and to improving health treatments and outcomes. We all know that the cost of America's health care is expensive. Is it worth the expense? We have to consider each of these advances before we make a blanket statement that we can't afford our current health care. If it's your life or your loved one's life we are referring to, can we afford it then? Never confuse the difference between cost or price and value.

11

HAVE I CONVINCED YOU YET?

In case I have not convinced you that the PPACA is a bloated, excessive piece of socialistic legislation that is bad for America and that the only reasonable action concerning this law is to repeal, let me try one more angle. A relatively new chart from the Center for Health Transformation is titled, "The New and Expanded Secretarial Powers in the Health Reform Law." This chart reveals the specifics of the HHS secretary's new responsibilities as revealed in the 2,562 pages of the PPACA.[1] Did you know that the new health reform law grants 1,968 powers to the HHS secretary? That's right, 1,968 powers.

The wording alone is disturbing, let alone the amount. The word "grants" makes it sound like a fairy godmother has appeared out of the sky and said, "Cinder-secretary, I'll grant you three—no, scratch that—I'll grant you 1,968 wishes—no, scratch that—powers." No unelected official has ever before received such power (1,968 powers, to be exact). And then there is the word "powers." It doesn't say "rules," "regulations," or "responsibilities"; it says "powers." When the word "powers" is used, it implies force or absolute authority. I have the "power" to shut your business down. I have the "power" to make you see more Medicare patients. I have the "power" to cut your reimbursement by 50 percent. Yes, Madame Secretary has 1,968 brand new "powers."

What is the HHS, where did it come from, and how long has it been around? In 1923, President Harding proposed the Department of Education and Welfare. Several presidents before him had tried to establish a similar department, but for various reasons his predecessors couldn't get this accomplished. The department was renamed the Department of Health and Human Services (HHS) in 1979 when its education functions were transferred to the newly created US Department of Education under the Department of Education Organization Act. The HHS was left in charge of the Social Security Administration, agencies comprising the US Public Health Service (PHS), and Family Support Administration. In 1995, Social Security was removed from the HHS and was established as an independent agency of the executive branch of the US government.[2]

The HHS is administered by the HHS secretary, who is appointed by the president with the advice and consent of the Senate. The PHS is the main division of the HHS and is led by the assistant secretary for Health. The Commissioned Corps of the PHS is led by the surgeon general. The Office of the Inspector General (OIG) investigates criminal activity for the HHS. Remember, the president has repeated several times that one of the ways in which America will pay for the PPACA is by recovering millions and millions of dollars in Medicare and Medicaid fraud and abuse. The OIG is one of the agencies for the 16,000 new federal agents who have been hired to police the health system.[3]

You will recall that health care makes up 17.3 percent of America's GDP, which means about $1 of every $5 is going to health care. Besides having control over the largest sector of the American economy, the HHS secretary now has an additional 1,968 powers granted to her. Matters of life and death for all Americans have just been handed over to one appointed bureaucrat. When Kathleen Sebelius was governor of Kansas, an article was published in one of the major national magazines that listed the ten most powerful and influential women in the nation;[4] Governor Sebelius was in the top four. I believe she has moved up to the undisputed number-one most powerful and influential woman in America today.

Should any nonelected bureaucrat have that much power? You probably think I'm exaggerating. She doesn't really have control over life-and-death matters facing every American, does she? Let's just see about that!

Here are just a few examples of the 1,968 new powers granted to the HHS secretary.

> Section 3307: Identification of Drugs in Certain Categories and Classes: (i) The secretary shall identify, as appropriate, categories and classes of drugs for which the secretary determines are of clinical concern. (ii) Criteria. The secretary shall use criteria established by the secretary in making any determination under subclause (I). (iii) Implementation. The secretary shall establish criteria … and any exceptions … through which the promulgation of a regulation which includes a public notice and comment period.[5]

If you sift through the legal jargon, the HHS secretary, with this one new power, will determine what drugs are appropriate for each clinical situation. This newly granted power establishes Kathleen Sebelius as the medication authority in America. The last time I checked, she was not a pharmacologist or a doctor. In fact, her credentials are that she was a previous insurance commissioner in Kansas. Does that qualify her as the medication expert? In reality, what this really allows the secretary to do is evaluate like medications and determine which drugs are affordable. Here we go again;

we will now allow a nonelected government official to tell us which medication will be paid for and therefore which medication works best for us. This is yet another example of one-size-fits-all medicine. Suppose you have cancer and are aware of three similar types of drugs appropriate for treatment. You know that one of these drugs works the best but is also the most expensive. Do you suppose that's the one that the secretary will approve? Or, more likely, do you suppose the secretary will select the cheapest drug of the three?

Worse yet, there are three cancer drugs (Drugs A, B, and C) available for your type of cancer, but the HHS secretary, with her newly granted medication power, determines that Drug A is most appropriate. You take Drug A for eight weeks, during which time your cancer spreads to another organ. Now, you and your doctor believe that you must quickly change to either Drug B or Drug C. However, when you go to the hospital to have Drug B for your chemotherapy, the pharmacist says, "Oh, I'm sorry, Drug B is not considered appropriate by the HHS secretary for your type of cancer. But you can always appeal this decision and ask for further review."[6]

Think of how long an appeal process will take. There are now between 18 and 34 million additional citizens who are receiving medical care. Government agencies have never been known for their swift action (except perhaps the IRS when you owe them back taxes). If this cancer is as aggressive as it sounds (spreading to a second organ in only eight weeks), this decision for your medication is now a matter of life and death. I can see this scenario: You fill out the appeal forms right then and there at the hospital, and you drop the forms in the mail on your way home. Ten weeks later, your cancer has spread with a vengeance and you die. The day of your funeral, a letter from the HHS comes to your home saying, "Your appeal has been received. Please complete the enclosed additional forms, and upon receipt we will notify you of the approximate length of time for which this appeal will take. Currently, our appeal process takes nine months. We hope this process has not cost you any inconvenience. Sincerely, the Secretary of the Department of Health and Human Services."

> Section 3310: Reducing Wasteful Dispensing of Outpatient Prescription Drugs in Long-Term Care Facilities: The secretary shall require PDP sponsors of prescription drug plans to utilize specific, uniform dispensing techniques, as determined by the secretary, in consultation with … any other stakeholders the secretary determines appropriate … when dispensing covered part D drugs to enrollees who reside in a long-term care facility in order to reduce waste associated with thirty-day refills.[7]

One of the problems that hospitals deal with every day is the cost associated with placing inpatients on their home medications during their hospital stay. The Food and Drug Administration (FDA) and the Drug Enforcement Administration (DEA) have strict regulations regarding dispensing a patient's home medication in the hospital. For example, mom is admitted to the hospital because she fell and broke her hip. She takes six medicines at home and one natural product (a fish-oil tablet) that she buys at the General Nutrition Centers store (known as GNC). The daughter brings all of mom's pill vials full of ninety days' worth of medication. Mom just happened to have her medication filled today before her accident. The daughter recently saw a friend's hospital bill that showed some unbelievable prices for her friend's medications while in the hospital. When she and her friend had discussed this, they concluded that the same medication that her friend took at home was at least four times more expensive in the hospital. The daughter recalled her friend saying she would be certain to bring her own medication with her the next time she was hospitalized, if at all possible, simply to save money.

The daughter, being a dutiful daughter and a conscientious taxpayer, remembered this and brings all of mom's home medicines. This presents a real problem in the hospital. The FDA and the

DEA are rigid and strict regarding administration of home medication, primarily because of the possibility of medication error. Who is responsible if the home medication happens to interact with the medicines being used on mom while she recovers from hip surgery? Then there's the problem of the daughter bringing the wrong medications from home, which is a legitimate concern if you have ever seen most people's medicine cabinets.

Well, the granted power of section 3310 listed above is specifically for long-term care facilities. Here's where this becomes an issue: To cut costs, Medicare has determined there is a formulary of a defined list of medications that they will cover during long-term assisted medical care. To save on cost, the daughter brings the ninety-day supply of the six medicines mom has been taking at home and presents them to the long-term facility where mom will be during her recovery from hip surgery. After the surgery, mom develops a complication of a joint infection, and the wound is left open to heal from the inside out, known as healing by secondary intention. The orthopedist suspects that mom will be in the long-term facility for at least eight weeks.

The daughter brings the bag of medications to the long-term facility and presents them to the admissions nurse. She evaluates every medication closely, gets out a list, and begins to sort the six medications. When she is finished, she hands four medicines back to the daughter and keeps two.

"Why are you giving these back to me?" the daughter inquires.

The nurse replies, "These two medicines are on the list, and these four medicines are not."

"What list?" the daughter asks.

"The list put out by the secretary of HHS. She decides which medications can be administered in the long-term facility." The nurse stops for a second, then says, "I'm sorry, I forgot, we can only take a thirty-day supply, and these are written for ninety days." She hands the two vials back to the daughter.

"Really?" the daughter asks. She begins to open up the vials and count a thirty-day supply.

However, the nurse stops her and says, "No, that won't work because it has to be a thirty-day prescription, and these bottles distinctly say ninety days."

"What about the fish oil I just bought at GNC?"

"Oh, sure, I take that, too. It's a great supplement, but it's not on the list."

"Really?" The daughter is perplexed. "What if I sneak it in?"

"You better be mighty careful, because if you are caught breaking the rules, Medicare or the secretary of the HHS can deny payment of any of this long-term stay. And that

could be as much as $60,000. It's about $1,200 to $1,500 a day here, depending on the home medication costs."

The daughter thinks it over. "If you would allow me to give you mom's home meds, I can help decrease the cost to the system."

"Oh, no, that's not allowed."

You can see how utterly ridiculous this becomes. Even when we have reasonable and logical ways to keep the costs down, we are not allowed to do so because of some rigid and inflexible rule and regulation established by a committee in Washington that possibly didn't even have any health providers on the board. Whenever the government tries to legislate the actual medical care, it doesn't work well.

Section 4102 (2): National Health and Nutrition Examination Survey: The secretary shall develop oral health care components that shall include tooth-level surveillance for inclusion in the National Health and Nutrition Examination Survey…the term "tooth-level surveillance" means a clinical examination where an examiner looks at each dental surface, on each tooth in the mouth and as defined by the Division of Oral Health of the CDC.[8]

The secretary is now an authority on dentistry. She has outlined the manner in which dental hygienists and dentist should do a "tooth-level surveillance" examination. Her level of expertise is quite clear when she was astute enough to point out "on each tooth in the mouth" as opposed to all those pesky little (and even big) teeth that pop up all over the body. There's nothing more alarming than to have a tooth found outside your mouth! I suspect this granted power actually has something to do with whether seniors will be able to have their dentures paid for by Medicare. I suspect the answer is "no." Why on earth does the secretary even have any oversight authority of the basic oral and tooth exam? This is yet another example of government intervention run amuck!

A book that has received significant attention is *The Road to Serfdom* by Friedrich August Hayek. He says, "The more the state plans, the more difficult planning becomes for the individual." These 1,968 granted powers and the 2,562 pages of the PPACA are excellent examples of this statement. After all, the more the state plans and grants special powers to one unelected bureaucrat, the fewer liberties and choices the average citizen has. This is why Socialism and big government don't work.

The granted-powers decree sounds more like something designed by a dictatorship or a monarch system rather than a republic. If you're thinking this is a bit extreme, consider these examples: Recently, Kathleen Sebelius made a series of threats to use one of these new 1,968 granted powers to punish health insurance companies who have dared to tell the truth about how health reform law has led to rate hikes for their customers. And to support the claim the HSS Secretary already has been granted way too much power in the health delivery arena, at the time of publication of this book, Kathleen Sebelius already had in access of 150,000 pages of regulations. Imagine the direct impact these regulations and restrictions will have upon our lives and on our health.

From the HHS, Kathleen Sebelius wrote:

"It has come to my attention that several health insurer carriers are sending letters to their enrollees falsely blaming premium increases for 2011 on the patient protections in the Affordable Care Act. I urge you to inform your members that there will be zero tolerance for this type of misinformation and unjustified rate increases…"

Then there are the many benefits that Secretary Sebelius is bestowing on her friends, thanks to her newly granted powers. In the *Wall Street Journal*, Karl Rove described how Secretary Sebelius granted a number of companies exemptions from key requirements in the PPACA. More than 33 percent of these employees are unionized compared with a mere 7 percent of the national work force.

On June 6, 2011, Congressman Tim Huelskamp addressed a letter to Secretary Sebelius in the name of transparency, fairness, and due process to have her explain her justification for her 1,372 special privilege exemptions or waivers that she granted to labor unions that have supported the president or to businesses that are in former speaker Pelosi's district.[9]

Wouldn't we all like an exemption from this health reform requirement? The specific language that grants the secretary this authority (part of these special powers she's been granted) states annual limit requirement waivers exempt recipients for one year from having to increase the amount of health care coverage they provide their workers. Each year between now and 2014, the maximum annual limit rises to a new, higher amount. Although the waivers are only for one year, recipients can reapply and be reappointed every year through 2014.

This is disturbing. If you have enough money, you can buy yourself a waiver or exemption from participating in the PPACA. I've already listed the previous groups that are exempt (Christian Scientists, Scientologists, Native Americans, illegal immigrants, and Muslims), and we can now add 1,372 unions and businesses to the list. Who will be left to pay for this bill? The answer may be the everyday, hard-working, tax-paying Americans who don't have the money or influence to purchase an exemption and who still maintain a level of scrupulousness that prevents them from lying and claiming they are Christian Scientists. This may actually be the easiest way to become a conscientious objector of health reform: Every tax-paying citizen declares him- or herself to be a Christian Scientist. Sure, you may actually have to attend a service or two, but it just may be financially worth it. I doubt the secretary will grant any of us everyday Americans an exemption? What do you think?

The other extremely disturbing problem with the secretary of the HHS having so much unilateral power is that she (or whoever is appointed to the position in the future) has the presidential authority to single-handedly ration health care. Of course, she will never call this "rationing of care," but any time the secretary or any of the boards or committees that oversee health care determines what treatment will be allowed, then they have the granted power to limit one's health treatment. This will always be under the guise of cost containment, but the reality is that behind every single medical therapy that is denied because of the overall cost of the treatment, there is a real live patient (at least for the moment, unless life-saving chemotherapy has just been denied) who has just been negatively affected by this limited medical therapy. This is why governments and politicians CANNOT legislate medicine. Once again, this is why one size does NOT fit all patients regarding their specific medical care.

12

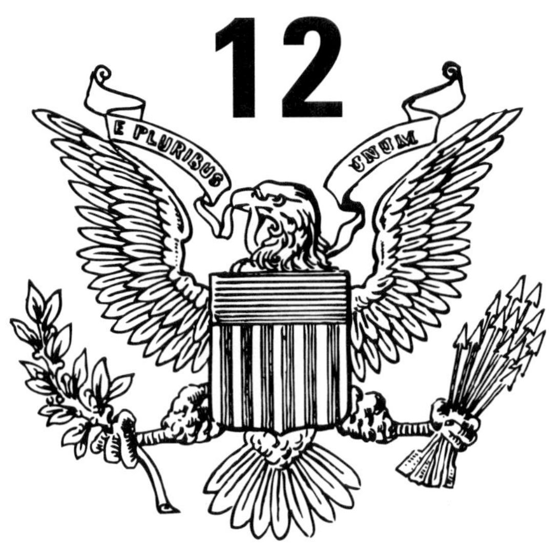

HOW WILL WE PAY FOR
THIS HEALTH REFORM BILL?

Margaret Thatcher said it best: "The problem with Socialists is they eventually run out of other people's money!"[1] According to the CBO, the PPACA will cost $938 billion between 2010 and 2019. Of course, using creative accounting measures, this paints a better picture than the real numbers. The PPACA was signed into law in March 2010, and we have already begun the process of starting to pay for this massive program. However, the actual health care to be provided under the health reform bill—that is, the actual health benefits that are to occur because of this legislation—don't begin until 2014. So, wouldn't a more accurate and a more honest accounting of the overall projected costs include those estimated expenses from 2014 until 2024? The CBO says when you look at the numbers for these ten years, the total expense is much greater at $2.5 trillion. There's a significant difference between $938 billion and $2.5 trillion—two and a half times more![2]

Using anyone's figures, this monstrosity is expensive! How can we afford it? Aren't Medicare and Social Security already under-funded? Haven't the president and the media been saying that Social Security checks won't be sent if we don't raise the debt ceiling? Regardless of one's political views or persuasions, we are over-spent as a nation. And now we are overspent as a health system.

There are many of the suggested methods we are going to try to use to pay for this. Several of these methods include; fines for Medicare fraud and abuse, and overall decrease in Medicare reimbursements, fines or penalties for those citizens and businesses who fail to obtain health insurance, a Medicare payroll tax, and a whole host of specialty taxes on such things as MRI's, CT's, and medical devices just to list a few.

Who do you think will carry the burden? The rich, right? Aren't they the deadbeats in this country, those evil rich who absolutely refuse to pay their share? Oh, that's right, the top 1 percent of earners in this country pay 95 percent of the tax burden. According to the Tax Foundation, the top 1 percent of earners consists of 1.4 million taxpayers, and they pay a larger share of the income tax burden than the bottom 134 million taxpayers combined. Let me say that in another way: If you took all the income taxes paid by the 134 million Americans who are the lower 99 percent based on their incomes and added them together, the total they paid in taxes would still be less than the total amount of taxes paid by the top 1 percent earners in America. That's right; 1 percent, or 1.4 million Americans (the haves, the evil rich, the group of people whom most of us workers in the lower and middle classes aspire to be) paid more in taxes than the other 134 million, or the other 99 percent earners, combined.[3] That is incomprehensible!

CLASS ENVY

Why are these people so vilified and so hated by everyone if they are carrying more than everyone else's fair share? Shouldn't we actually be thanking them and holding them in high regards instead of bad-mouthing them? What's even crazier is that anyone who has a work ethic at all aspires to achieve their level of success. We all say that money isn't everything, but it would be fun to see what it's like for a while. How have the so-called spokespersons for this country been allowed or able to reframe the discussion so that nearly everyone in America despises the wealthy? While we are discussing the rich, have you ever wondered why many of our Congressmen and -women arrive in Washington as upper middle class, well off but not rich by today's standards, and when they leave Washington (way too many terms later) they are all millionaires? How does that happen?

We have decided to use Robin Hood as our social hero; he takes from the rich and gives to the poor. As a kid, I thought Robin Hood was pretty darn cool. In the movies he was always the hero, he always got the girl, and the rich people were always portrayed as arrogant and greedy. It was easy to despise this group of people, based on Hollywood's presentation. Of course, I never thought about it much as a kid, but in Robin Hood's day, of serfdom, you were either born rich or born poor. There didn't seem to be a whole lot of opportunities to move from the poor class to the wealthy. The problem is, most people don't ever really ponder why the Robin Hood philosophy worked in the Dark Ages. Instead, they're happy to demonize the wealthy and run with the concept of taking from the rich and giving to the poor.

Having been fortunate enough to be born and raised in America in the twentieth century and now living in the twenty-first century, I completely disagree with the take-from-the-rich-and-give-to-the-poor motto. In fact, many of the rich in America worked long and hard to become wealthy after being poor for many years. That's what makes our country so great and completely different from the days of Robin Hood; we can move from one economic class to another. There are many opportunities for us to make money in America. Therefore, we shouldn't have any need to confiscate the wealthy citizens' money and redistribute it to the less fortunate and poor of our society. Unfortunately, getting that through our now-socialistic Congress's heads is much harder than it should be. The social justice movement is misguided and harmful to the principles that made our republic great. We need to abandon our Robin Hood principles and let all citizens assume responsibility for their own finances, their own health insurance, and their own lives. The nanny-state philosophy does only one thing: It creates more dependents who need a nanny.

Did you know that Benjamin Franklin, one of our exceptional founding fathers, looked at America as a company? He said that each individual citizen is a stockholder of the United States. One of his suggestions was logical and made a lot of sense (however, if any influential leader in our country were to ever suggest it, the government just might bring back the old public punishment of tar and feathering): Only the people who have invested in the company—the financial stakeholders—should have a say in how the company is run. Following this line of thinking, we could issue a stock certificate to all American citizens when they are born or to people who become naturalized citizens. But this certificate would not entitle them to voting rights, as they have not paid into the government coffers yet. When American citizens reach the age of eighteen years and have gained employment, they would be able to vote. This isn't too different from our current system, right? Here's the caveat: Citizens after the age of eighteen years would have the right to vote only if they were taxpayers. They would have to be the people footing the bills to make our country run. Sure, all those folks who are not taxpayers would not like this idea. But think about it; the people in a company who help make decisions are the actual investors. If you are on the take, or if you are on the receipt rather than being a contributor or a taxpayer, then why should you have any say in how the money is spent? You would be a stockholder if you were an American citizen, and you would become a voting member if you were a productive member of society. Once you would begin to make some money and pay taxes, you could assume a voting role. This would solve the illegal immigrant problem. It would also help persuade the members of Congress, who decide how they will vote on legislation, to not make their decisions according to how many votes this will get them or which group of citizens they can gain favor with. Instead, we would begin to run the government and, in turn, America as if it were a company or a corporation. I think Benjamin Franklin may have had something here. If you disagree, then would you support a flat tax, where all citizens participated in paying taxes, even if it were only a pittance regarding the poor?[4]

TAXES, TAXES, AND MORE TAXES

Here are many of the taxes, some of which are already being imposed:

Beginning in 2013, individuals who earn $200,000 or more, and couples who make $250,000 or more, will see an increase in their Medicare tax. Remember, for those who work for an employer, the employer withholds 1.45 percent of their salary and sends this to Washington on the employees' behalf every pay period. (Take a long hard look at your paycheck stub and study it closely.) This is the Medicare part A tax. This contribution that you have been making since you joined the working class helps pay all our seniors' Medicare expenses. They paid in during their working years, too. Guess what? This 1.45 percent just went up to 2.35 percent.[5]

Starting in 2012, the Medicare payroll tax will be expanded to include unearned income. This is a 3.8 percent tax on investment proceeds from partnerships, royalties, and rents for families making $250,000 or more and individuals making $200,000 or more. That means that any of your investments that return anything are now considered "unearned" income.[6] Let me see if I get this: I decide to venture into the rental business. I buy a couple of dilapidated Department of Housing and Urban Development houses that were recently foreclosed. I'm fortunate and obtain them for a decent price. I want to be a good landlord, so I take $10,000 and invest that in my property. I reshingle the roofs, repair the siding, replace the carpeting and tiles, paint the walls, and repair the pipes. I do the work myself to keep my expenses down. I also have just enough of my $10,000 to buy nicer, used furnaces. I do this for both homes for $40,000 per house ($80,000 total) and $10,000 repair expenses per house ($20,000 total) for a total investment of $100,000. I'm fortunate to locate two families who are in need of renting a home. It's a landlord's market right now, and many people are renting. I charge $1,400 per house for a total of $2,400 per month for both houses or a total of $28,800 per year in rent money. My accountant says I have $1,000 of expenses per month with each house when he takes into consideration the initial investment as well as the standard depreciation. My total deductible expense for both houses for one year is $24,000. Thus, my net earnings are $28,800 minus $24,000, or $4,800. Let's say that I'm married, and together my wife and I make $250,000. This means that, according to our government, I have $4,800 of "unearned" investment (rent) money. First, to call this hard work I engaged in to make this investment happen "unearned" is insulting. Why is it declared "unearned?" If you want to declare something unearned, declare the annual raises that Congress gives themselves that push the envelope every time regarding cost of living and inflationary increases. The rest of us in the working world are fortunate if we receive one-fourth of a cost of living increase in our salaries; in my experience, it just doesn't happen every year. My $4,800 unearned income will now be taxed (starting in 2012) at 3.8 percent for a total of $182.40 that I now owe to the federal government.

What about other investments? How about precious metals? If you happened to buy gold or silver when they were at $600 or $12 an ounce, respectively, and now they are worth three times your investment, your good decision is unearned, according to Uncle Sam. In other words, you did nothing to earn it. The name of this tax implies you had this investment income dropped in your lap. Keep in mind that this unearned tax is on top of all your other taxes, like your capital gains tax and your income tax and, under the right circumstances, your estate tax. Because you are being forced to pay this tax on your investment, you should be able to get reimbursed 3.8 percent for your loss if you happen to make a bad investment and lose money, correct? I don't think so! This doesn't provide much incentive to invest in America. So much for having an entrepreneurial spirit.

Insurance companies will have to pay their share. Starting in 2011 until 2018, they will pay an estimated $47.5 billion in new taxes. In 2018, it is estimated that they will pay at least $14.3 billion a year.[7] They should pay their share, right? Do you think they'll simply say that this is their own personal responsibility and therefore cinch up their belts and pay out the nose? Would you if you were running an insurance company? Of course not. Insurance companies, like any business, will do everything they can to pass this expense on to the client. This, in turn, will lead to an overall increase in health insurance costs and specifically in premiums. But I thought the current administration said that our health insurance costs and the overall expenses associated with health care would go down. It doesn't look that way to me.

There is now a 10 percent tax on tanning salons. This is a federal excise tax that started on July 1, 2010.[8] You see, everyone will get to share in paying for the PPACA, but why tanning salons? Is it because they're supposed to be bad for your skin? Is that why they must pay? Why not tax fast food or candy shops? Shouldn't these merchants be singled out just like the tanning salon owners? The total revenue from tanning salon taxes is estimated to be $2.5 billion over the next decade. I would suspect that this egregious tanning tax may put many of these tanning salons out of business. Does it ever make you wonder if the current administration dislikes small business owners?

Then there's the pharmaceutical industry. Remember, these companies are dastardly wealthy and must be punished for all their greed. Granted, drug companies have strong balance sheets and favorable profit and loss columns, but do they bring us anything of value? Of course they do. Look at all the invaluable medications that have changed the entire landscape of the medical system over the past forty years, such as amazing advances in oncology, unbelievable breakthroughs in cardiology, and infectious disease research that has allowed our citizens to live a reasonable quality of life with HIV. All these advances have happened because of the research-and-development commitment from these pharmaceutical industries. The pharmaceutical manufacturer tax is estimated at a collection of $16.7 billion from now until 2019 and $2.8 billion each year afterward, not to mention the current taxes the manufacturers already pay.[9] Do you think that the drug companies will eat all this cost? I doubt it. Like the insurance companies, they'll pass this on to the consumer. Medication costs will go up, and continued emphasis on research will go down. I predict if the PPACA health bill is not repealed that we will enter a long dry period in which the medical advances will significantly diminish. The real breakthroughs come from the private sector, and where's their incentive to continue to produce new and amazing products? It went by the wayside with the stroke of the president's pen. Edward Bulwer-Lytton was indeed correct, the pen is mighty than the sword![10]

Next, there are the medical device companies. These are the companies that make devices such as pacemakers (recall that the president said on his health reform tour that grandma would not qualify for the pacemaker but would instead be given a pill[11] ... I wonder if Michelle Obama's mother were to ever need a pacemaker if she would be granted the medicine instead...), orthotics, prosthetics, and infusaports for intravenous medication and insulin pumps. The taxes will affect such services as CT scans, MRI scans, blood pressure cuffs, and surgical instruments. The companies will pay a 2.3 percent excise tax and the projected total tax revenue of $2 billion each year. These particular taxes are expected to increase health insurance premiums for a family of four by $1,000 a year.[12] One would think that because these device companies develop some of the most important life-saving pieces of medical equipment— which, in turn, improve the patients' quality of life and ultimately lead to a significant decrease in the cumulative medical expenses for each individual patient—that the government would develop an economic incentive program to encourage their research-and-development efforts instead of taxing these companies. That's how the free market and the private sector work.

Unfortunately, this goes directly against the principles of big intrusive government. Who will ultimately pay for these taxes? That's right, the cost will be passed on to the consumer.

Businesses begin a brand new era starting in 2012. All businesses must submit a 1099 form every time they spend at least $600.[13] Before the PPACA became law, businesses were required to complete the 1099 form only when they made a payment to independent contractors. Any purchase over $600 will now be taxable. Your local mom-and-pop computer-repair shop will now have to fill out a 1099 form every time they purchase anything over $600, including office supplies, computer supplies, software, books, and so on. The volume of paperwork (which was already onerous) just went up exponentially. I can't fathom why anyone would want to go into private business any more. Where will our youth find their jobs in the future? I suppose the only safe haven at all is to work for the state. That makes sense; almost every one of the new jobs President Obama has claimed to have created has come directly from the government. And remember, the state employee makes on average $70,000, whereas the private sector employee makes nearly $30,000. But our health care costs will go down!

Don't forget the Cadillac health plans. Any health plan once known as a Cadillac plan that costs the individual $10,200 and the family $27,500 or more will now be taxed at a whopping 40 percent rate. This tax begins in 2018 and is expected to bring in $32 billion.[14] (In case you're wondering why this particular tax doesn't happen until 2018, it's the bargaining chip the administration threw to the union leaders.) If you were previously able to afford such health plans, this will be all the more difficult from 2018 onward. Another caveat concerning this type of tax is that it isn't adjusted for inflation. The IRS uses the term "bracket creep," in which inflation over time gradually drives you into a higher tax bracket. That's what will happen with these higher-dollar Cadillac plans if the PPACA isn't repealed. Sooner or later, in one to three decades, your employer-sponsored tax plan (which, over time, will cost what a Cadillac plan costs today but in tomorrow's inflationary dollars will not be worth a Cadillac plan based on services) will one day be subject to the 40 percent tax.

One of the most blatant taxes that will go into effect in 2013 affects all Americans who have a flexible spending account (FSA). Currently, about 16 million Americans use pretax dollars to purchase medical services and medical supplies. In 2013, the amount of money that can be set aside for health services will be cut in half from $5,000 to $2,500.[15] These pretax dollars have provided these 16 million Americans and their families with such things as dental care, orthodontic care, eyeglasses, medication copayments, over-the-counter medicines, insurance deductibles, Band-Aids, and even some cosmetic procedures. To make this even worse, already in 2011, the FSA pretax dollars are not allowed to be used for over-the-counter medications. But Mr. President, you said this new bill was about each American getting affordable health care. How does cutting this program benefit me and my fellow citizens?

You can see the tax man cometh, and the tax man will taketh away! You can also see how much of these taxes and expenses to companies will be passed right on down the chain to you, the consumer. It appears that these far-reaching taxes will have a detrimental effect on the health insurance prices, ultimately leading to an increase in the cost of health care and health insurance. Then there's the increase in everyone's taxes. Conservative numbers suggest that all these taxes will result in an increase in taxes for the highest income earners by $52,000 a year, and those income earners in the lowest tax bracket can expect to see an increase in their taxes by an estimated $2,000 a year. Christian Science sounds better all the time.

13

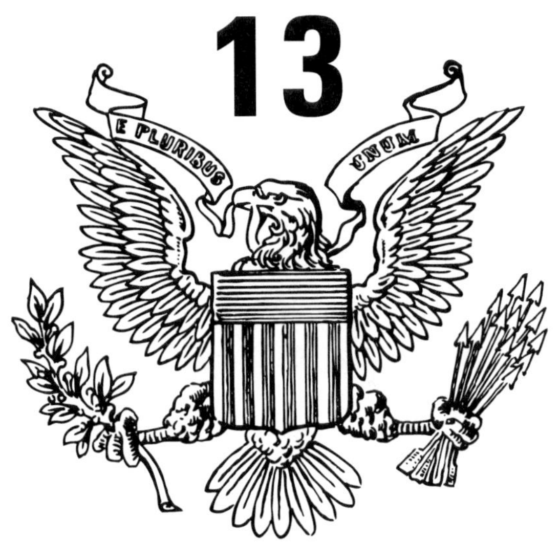

THE SYSTEM REALLY IS BROKEN.

My sister recently told me her experience with a nosebleed, of all things, that she developed on a typical Sunday morning. A persistent nosebleed can actually become a serious problem if the bleeding cannot be stopped. She tried all the standard treatments, like pressure on the bridge of her nose, ice to her nose, tissue in her nostril, lying on her back, standing upright, and hopping up and down on one leg in a circle for ten minutes (that one was my idea just to see if she would do anything that a doctor suggested!), but none of these treatments worked. After six hours of bleeding with no end in sight, she finally reluctantly agreed to go to the emergency department. Upon arrival, and after the emergency department personnel realized she legitimately could not get her nose to stop bleeding, she was escorted to an examination room. Within minutes, a PA appeared, examined her, and then attempted to cauterize the bleeding vessel with a silver nitrate stick. This attempt at treatment failed. The PA then placed a nasal tampon in the back of her nostril and inflated the small balloon (not so small, according to my sister). With the balloon inflated, the bleeding successfully stopped because of the pressure placed on the small injured vessel. After observing her for about thirty minutes to be certain that the bleeding was under control, the personnel discharged my sister. The nosebleed successfully healed over time. My sister is a single teacher who makes an average teacher's salary, but the soreness she felt in her pocketbook has not yet healed. A few weeks later, she received a $4,800 bill from the emergency department. Of this bill, $1,200 went to the doctor. She told me that the doctor came into the examination room for about ten seconds; never examined her; simply said, "Looks like everything's under control"; and then abruptly left.

These are the most common frustrations I hear from patients a couple of times a week. They can't believe that anyone should make $1,200 for ten seconds of work. They can't believe that the doctor can even legally bill for not even examining the patient. They also have a difficult time with the hospital and the emergency department billing $3,600 ($4,800 total bill minus the $1,200 doctor's bill) for forty-five to sixty minutes of treatment. When I hear these stories, I have to agree that the patients have a valid point. I am in total agreement that many key elements to our system are broken. I recently heard a friend of mine, Dr. Jeff Lawhead, an FP, describe that we don't have a health delivery crisis but rather a health insurance crisis. Thinking about this, I believe he is exactly correct. In my sister's example, this also looks like a health insurance problem more so than a health delivery problem. She will tell you that the health care she received was entirely appropriate. Her beefs are about the overall cost and that the doctor could step in the room, speak for a couple of seconds, leave without examining her, and bill her $1,200. Her beefs are valid.

The doctor should not have done that. He placed his full trust in the PA and made the judgment that the PA had handled things appropriately. He could have taken a bit more time, and it would have made my sister feel better about him. However, his argument would be that she came in for a nosebleed, it was handled appropriately, and why did he need to put on a show simply to make her feel good about him? One can see that explanation, as well.

Let's break this down further. The doctor will not take home $1,200. The PA probably works for the doctor and will receive his salary from him and his group. There are overhead expenses for this bill, such as salaries, benefits (including health insurance), malpractice insurance, billing, and probably transcription. Does that warrant a $1,200 bill? Probably not. But the care was administered by the PA. So, what was this visit worth? If my sister had paid in cash because she bartered, shopped around, and found the best price, what would be the reasonable fee? $250? $500? It's probably somewhere in that ballpark of $500.00. So, why can the doctor bill three and four times that total? Here's the problem: Medicaid, Medicare, and many poor health insurance companies would have paid only $50 to $75 total for the PA's forty-five to sixty minutes of time. Because the poor payers pay such a pittance, the doctor charges a higher rate; therefore, when the client has quality insurance, this insurance company's payment will offset the other five patients who had ineffective insurance in which the doctor and his group actually lost money. That's right, the good insurance companies and the self-payers who use cash are paying significantly higher fees than the rest of the insurances and public plans like Medicaid and Medicare.[1] I thought the doctor must charge the same price for each different service. I thought he couldn't charge a different rate based on what type of insurance the patient had. That is correct. But charging and collecting are two different things. The doctor has set his fee higher so that when he receives payment from Medicare and he's forced to accept whatever Medicare pays (no matter what he billed to Medicare), he makes up the difference from the better insurance companies.

The same explanation applies to the hospitals, except for one additional item: They have a powerful and influential lobbying group known as the American Hospital Association (AHA). The AHA has been able to influence Medicare reimbursement and, for that matter, any insurance carrier reimbursement to the point that any hospital service gets significantly higher reimbursement than the same service in an outpatient facility. When a payment from Medicare is decided for a particular service, and if it's a hospital-based service, the CMS calculates the hospital based payment for routine care at cost times 2.5[2]. Hospital reimbursement is generally two and a half times higher than the same service (at minimum) performed in an outpatient facility.

For example, a patient has an MRI study of the shoulder at an outpatient diagnostic center. The cost is $500 for the study. The same patient has an MRI of the shoulder at a hospital, and the cost of the study is $2,500. How can that be? Well, hospitals have higher overhead; they deal with higher levels of acuity and need greater levels of care. Therefore, their overall costs are higher.[3] Why wouldn't the public demand to have all their ambulatory exams done in an outpatient facility? The answer is multifaceted. First, the patients are not informed to the point of understanding that the outpatient facility has the cheaper prices. Second, the doctors are not as informed as they should be or they have grown weary of dealing with the levels of red tape they have to go through to get the outpatient exam preauthorized by the insurance company. Also, if the insurance company denies payment, the doctors don't want to incur the wrath of their patients, so they toss up their hands and say, "Go wherever your insurance wants you to." Third, the government has stepped in and made it almost impossible for doctors to have any ownership in ancillary medical facilities (known as a Stark violation). The doctors are therefore jaded from the government insistence at limiting what they can and can't do, so they give in and say again, "Go wherever your insurance wants you to." Fourth, the

AHA has aided hospitals significantly regarding reimbursement, so doctors simply let that go and refuse to fight the system anymore. Lastly, insurance companies have dictated what services can be done when and where. As a result, doctors are tired of battling with insurance. This is a laborious and never-ending process to try to ensure that insurance will pay for the appropriate procedure or medical test, and the appeal process generally lies at the doctors' feet. Doctors didn't pursue medicine to have to fight administrative battles with insurance. They didn't pursue medicine to fill out reams of forms and documents. They didn't pursue medicine to always have someone, generally much less educated in medicine, looking over their shoulders and telling them how to practice medicine. They pursued medicine to take care of people and to practice their trade. Despite public perception, most doctors are very good at being doctors, finding the medical problem, and offering a reasonable treatment plan for their patients.

There's one other problem that has developed as a direct result of doctors overcharging insurance and self-payers to make up the difference for all those companies and for the CMS when the reimbursement is next to nothing: The government stepped in and tried to regulate the health insurance industry. The Nixon administration created the Health Maintenance Organization (HMO) in 1971 in an attempt to keep health costs down, and the Health Maintenance Act of 1973[4] passed Congress. The new law included numerous regulations to encourage businesses to turn to HMOs for their employees' medical care. Companies with more than twenty-five workers were required to offer at least one HMO as an option for health insurance. These HMOs became unpopular by the early 2000s because they were too aggressive at cost cutting. However, what happened as a result of the HMOs was that the government had now positioned itself to mandate greater requirements and regulations to both providers and insurance companies. If a physician signed up as a provider for a certain health insurance company, the physician was agreeing to accept whatever payment for medical services rendered that the insurance determined to pay. The government was more than happy to step back and let these particular insurance companies themselves work out their pay scales with the doctors. Doctors still feel the ill effects of several of these insurance companies. An excellent example of this type of less-than-favorable pay scale is a particular company for whom I am one of their network radiologists. What this means is that I have agreed to accept whatever payment they deem appropriate for whatever radiological exam I perform. Generally, I receive about $22 to $25 from most insurance companies for an interpretation of a chest x-ray. On a rare occasion I may receive $30. Our group charges $44 to interpret a chest x-ray, knowing that we will usually receive less than $44 from the majority of insurance companies. On the bottom of the check that I recently received for this service was a statement saying, "As a network provider, you have agreed to accept the payment that we approve for this service. You cannot bill the remainder of your fee to the patient." The check was for $1.38. There are few products or services in this world that I could get for $1.38.[5]

The real kicker is that I assume the liability for reading this exam for a measly $1.38. These are real examples of some of the many problems that occur when the government decides to regulate the health insurance industry.

Yes, the system is broken, without a doubt, but why not look at the areas that are broken, improve them, and then maintain those areas that are already functioning well? Instead, we've turned to the federal government for our solutions, and that's a scary option. I can't think of one department that the government runs efficiently. Can you?

14

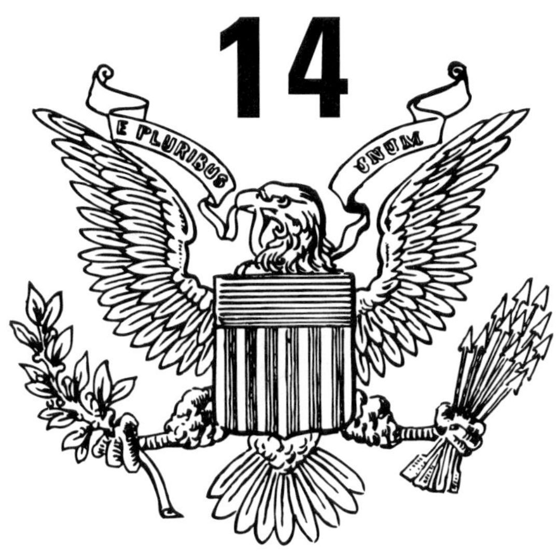

LONG-TERM CARE SCHEME

As I've repeated a couple of times now, one of the more infuriating things about the PPACA is the continual desire to quietly sneak a bad idea past the general public while the public have their heads turned toward their own busy, everyday lives. The best example of this deception and lack of transparency is the Community Living Assistance Services and Support (CLASS) Act, tucked neatly away in the middle of the massive 2,562 pages of the bill. Kent Conrad (D-ND), who actually voted in favor of the bill, described the CLASS Act as "a Ponzi scheme of the first order, the kind of thing that Bernie Madoff would have been proud of." The bill could not have been more inaccurately named. The acronym CLASS-LESS would have been the best description.[1]

Medicare does not pay for long-term care. It's estimated that twelve million Americans over the age of sixty-five will need long-term care by 2020.[2] Long-term care includes those services that many elderly, chronically ill, or disabled people need to perform their activities of daily living, like getting dressed, feeding themselves, performing basic hygiene and bathing, and using the bathroom. We usually assume that long-term care means the patient is in a nursing home; however, today, many of these services are provided by health professionals who deliver the care at the patients' homes. Long-term care can include nursing home care, assisted living care, or home health care.

Because a number of Medicare recipients will need this service, the government has elected to enter into the business of providing long-term care. An easy solution would have been to provide real financial incentives to purchase private coverage. Instead, the government leaders chose to create an entirely new social program, the CLASS program.

Starting in 2011, provided the HHS secretary can complete the appropriate regulations for the CLASS program, employers who unilaterally decide they will participate in the program will automatically enroll all their employees unless the employees formally opt out. Between $150 and $240 in long-term (CLASS) premiums will be deducted from their paychecks every month.

The participants will receive from $50 to $100 a day if they become disabled, provided that they are unable to perform at least two activities of daily living. To qualify for cash payouts, the participants must have paid premiums for at least five years before drawing benefits.[3]

The CBO estimates that the program's first ten years will lower the federal deficit by $72 billion through 2019.[4] However, to say that the program will bring in revenue is completely misleading because no cash outlay can occur for the first five years of contribution, for each person must have paid in for five years. Counting ten years of premiums against five years of payouts makes it easy to show that the program is financially sound in the first decade. Once again, we're dealing with shady accounting, or fuzzy math. Of course, the CLASS program will look profitable if the first five years of collecting premiums each month are untouched. But once the five years are met, the amount of money potentially going out far exceeds the amount coming in. Long-term care is expensive. To tout this program as yet another program that will help decrease the federal budget is disingenuous.

The CBO's long-term projection of the CLASS program estimates that the program will pay out more than it takes in by 2025, and by 2035 the CLASS program will have increased the budget deficit by tens of billions of dollars each decade. Even Secretary Sebelius, when placed under oath by the Senate Finance Committee, admitted that the CLASS Act was totally unsustainable.[5]

Senate Finance Committee Chairman Max Baucus (D-MT) stated on the Senate floor, "I am no fan of the CLASS Act myself." As I mentioned earlier, Senator Kent Conrad (D-ND) declared the CLASS program a Ponzi scheme.[6] If that is really how you feel about this legislation, senators, then why did you vote for it? This is yet another reason why Congress should stay out of the health care business; they often know the right thing to do but, because of their own personal and political agendas, are incapable of doing it. No wonder the country is broke. No wonder we have a health insurance crisis!

The health insurance system may be broken, and even the health delivery system has some problems, but the design of our American government is not broken. When America is informed, and when everyday citizens get involved, positive things can happen. For example, in April 2011, US Senator John Thune (R-SD) and US Representative Charles Boustany, Jr., MD (R-Southwest Louisiana) introduced S 720 and HR 1173, bills to repeal the CLASS Act.[7] There was significant public outcry regarding the poor structure and unsustainable expense of this long-term care entitlement program buried within the PPACA.

This should serve as an excellent example for how to deal with each of the expensive and intrusive parts of the PPACA. It is possible to put a stop to any individual piece of the legislation or to scrap the entire bill and start over, focusing on numerous effective areas of our current health and insurance systems and repairing their many broken areas. If, after reading each chapter leading up to this, you find yourself frustrated, discouraged, and overwhelmed and believing there is no way to stop the massive intrusion of the PPACA (because it already the law of the land), I understand. However, your belief that we cannot stop this legislation from taking over our health system is incorrect. Senator Thune and Representative Boustany have just given us an excellent example how we can reverse the current direction. This won't be easy; the PPACA looks like a twenty-ton freight train barreling down directly at the current health system, including the patients, providers, and insurance carriers. But we can stop this train, derail a portion or all of it, and take the old freight train that has a great deal of usefulness left in it, retool it, repair it, fix the many problems, and send it on down the track. The only way to do this is to repeal each individual part of the PPACA, methodically, step by step, one piece of counter legislation at a time. Or, a quicker and probably easier approach would be to repeal the entire PPACA in one fell swoop. Either way, this can be done. All of us who realize just how inept this law is must demand this from Congress. Pick up a pen and paper, or sit down at your keyboard with your word processor, or pick up your telephone and tell your congressperson your opinion of the PPACA. Do it right now; don't delay. What are you waiting for? I realize that you, like most of us, don't believe that an individual can make a difference, but collectively we can make a difference when we all speak up. You can make a difference because even with all their rhetoric and their personal and political agendas, members of Congress like being in Washington—to stay there, they all need each of our votes. Our individual votes are our only bargaining chips, our only negotiating tools. So, contact your congressperson right now. We need a large public outcry to derail this train.

One of the "hot topics" in health care reform over the past two years is "accountable care organizations", the ACO's. In response to the PPCACA suggestion that ACO's be offered, private insurance has responded with currently 13 ACO's offered throughout the country. More ACO's are currently in the works.

What is an ACO? In order to understand an ACO, you need look no further than the name, *accountable* care organization. These organizations have been developed to address the accelerated costs in medicine by holding the providers accountable. That's how ACO's got their name. These organizations came about specifically to hold the provider accountable for their patient's outcomes and for the overall cost of health care. In other words, this is similar to incentive pay, or payment rendered based on specific outcome. The clinician is held accountable or responsible for how the patient responds to the specific medical treatment. This health care organization is a combination of several previous attempted organizations, like Health Maintenance Organizations (HMO's), and Preferred Provider Organizations (PPO's), as well as Diagnostic Related Groups (DRG'S).

For example, let's say that a forty year old patient develops pneumonia. And let's presume that this patient, Mr. Smith, sees Dr. Jones, who is a member of an ACO. Dr. Jones examines Mr. Smith and decides based on physical examination, that Mr. Smith probably has pneumonia. He determines this based on Mr. Smith's vital signs (increased respiratory rate, and elevated temperature) as well as his physical examination (crackles in the lung base on auscultation). As Dr. Jones is a provider in an ACO, he will be paid his fees for caring for Mr. Smith based on Mr. Smith's response to Dr. Jones's prescribed treatment. If Dr. Jones gets the diagnosis right, especially on the first attempt, he will receive maximum payment for his services. In this way, ACO's are incentive based. Dr. Jones has incentive to be the best doctor he can be. The less money he spends making the diagnosis, the better. [8]

And, in this respect, ACO's are similar to the DRG's that we already have tried and still use to some extent. DRG's were initially designed to assign a specific fee to each of the many hospital based medical services available to the general public. With DRG's there is an average fee for treating a specific condition. For example, if a patient has gall stones and needs their gallbladder removed, using the DRG method of payment, CMS studied the average expense for admission to the hospital, having surgery to remove the gallbladder, and all post-operative care including medication. CMS also took into consideration the cost of living and the standard of care in each part of the country. Then, they assigned a flat average fee for having one's gallbladder removed, from start to finish. In a perfect world, using the DRG method, for any gallbladder surgery and post-operative care, the surgeons are paid the same for care and treatment of this specific patient and disease, and the hospitals are paid a flat fee for the same care centered around the gallbladder surgery and the patient's post operative care. The total costs are determined by calculating an average of all gallbladder surgeries, taking into consideration the cost-of-living in the particular part of the country where the surgery is performed.

When this DRG system was developed, the doctors were told that this would solve our cost issues. And that this would mandate how much all doctors were paid based on their outcomes. However, one major problem occurred, patients and diseases didn't always follow the textbooks or the predicted outcomes. Sometimes complications do occur. And sometimes it takes longer for one patient to recuperate from gallbladder surgery than another. And when this happened, the system failed.

If the average stay in the hospital following gallbladder surgery was twenty-four hours, then the physician was expected to send their patient home in twenty-four hours, regardless of whether or not their patient followed the average and the expected outcome. And in turn, they would receive the average payment for this service, regardless of how long the patient actually needed care. As you might imagine, this system worked part of the time, provided the patient followed the predicted outcome. But, if the patient's outcome varied at all, and the patient needed more care, the cost of care provided after the twenty-four hour window was not paid for.

The idea behind the DRG was to provide the doctors with incentives to remain within the standard of care for each specific disease and the appropriate treatment. In this respect, ACO's and DRG's have some similarities. Yet, once again, doctors take the brunt of the criticism. Using the name "Accountable" Care Organization in and of its self, suggests that doctors are currently not held accountable, and therefore need a system that mandates accountability. I'd suggest that this premise is wrong from the start. Doctors are held accountable. It's called medical malpractice, and medical litigation for medical negligence. It's also known as the Board of Healing Arts, the governing body of health professionals in each state. When a doctor practices outside the standard of care, they are required to return to the practice of medicine that is within the acceptable standard as outlined by their governing Board of Healing Arts, or they end up having poor patient outcomes that ultimately leads to litigation and medical malpractice cases. In either situation, the physicians currently are already held accountable. So, the name alone begins with a false premise.

What makes an ACO different than a DRG is that the incentive pay for the care and services provided is not determined as a blanket average. In an improvement from the DRG, the ACO determines payment for medical care rendered based on individual outcome, not on averages. For example, let's continue our discussion of Mr. Smith with pneumonia, and Dr. Jones. Dr. Jones, practicing within the confines of the ACO, has accepted that he will receive his remuneration for the care he provides for Mr. Smith's pneumonia, based on how cost effective he can diagnosis and treat the pneumonia, and based on the accuracy of his treatment. If Dr. Jones is a high level physician, like all of us are expected to be (yes, we are already held accountable to a current standard), then Dr. Jones will practice evidenced based medicine. He will treat each patient individually. He won't get wrapped up in averages. His only concern will be how he makes the correct diagnosis, in the most cost effective manner. If Mr. Smith's findings on examination convince Dr. Jones that the correct diagnosis is pneumonia, and if Dr. Jones feels certain of this diagnosis without the need to order any additional diagnostic tests, then Dr. Jones will be financially rewarded for his accuracy and his cost effective method of diagnosis and treatment, provided that his diagnosis was indeed correct and provided that Mr. Smith responds to Dr. Jones's treatment. However, if Dr. Jones could not definitively make a diagnosis based on the examination alone, and he determined that Mr. Smith needed a chest x-ray, or even a CT scan to make the diagnosis, then he would still be reimbursed for the overall care he provided Mr. Smith, just at a lower fee schedule.

The other important philosophical component of the ACO is that physicians become overall managers of patient's health care. Instead of caring for patients using a reactive treatment approach, doctors are encouraged, and financially rewarded for taking a pro-active and a preventative approach to patient health care. Using the ACO model, physicians become general managers of each of their individual patient's health care. The focus is on healthy living, preventative care, and proactive engaging medicine. On first glance, this all sounds pretty good. Wouldn't doctors like all of their patients to start off healthy? The main problem with this is that many times patients don't want to be that healthy. When your doctor says, quit eating fast food, quit smoking, lose thirty pounds, and start exercising thirty minutes five days a week, how many of us run right out and start doing this. Your doctor wasn't kidding when they made those specific recommendations. But, suggesting and requiring are two different things. If the doctor gets reimbursed based on outcomes, should the doctor be penalized when the patient doesn't comply or produce results? Or should the doctor be allowed to fire the patient from the practice if and when it becomes apparent that the patient's lack of attention to their health and well-being is ultimately costing the doctor money. Let doctors begin firing patients for healthy lifestyle reasons and I think we'll have an even bigger problem on our hands than the many complex issues already facing our health system.

In some respects, the ACO sounds like it could work. Unfortunately, there are many more plausible reasons why it will likely fail. First and foremost, the patient does not always follow the textbook. And so, no matter how skilled the doctor, how astute the diagnostician, or how experienced the clinician, doctors will not get it right every time. And, even more importantly, doctors will not get it right the first time, with each and every patient. Diseases do not always follow the predicted outcomes. With ACO's, the clinician gets punished when the patient and the disease do not follow the usual or predicted outcome.

And, of even greater concern, the only way that doctors have the freedom and comfort to follow their experiences and convictions to not order additional diagnostic studies is if we first enact or implement overall medico-legal tort reform. But, as I've already pointed out, no such discussion is occurring throughout the halls of Congress. Until America gets serious about tort reform, ACO's will not work.

Finally, one of the other problems facing the ACO is who gets to determine the fee schedule. And how do they decide what each treatment should be worth. Why should treating pneumonia without ordering a chest x-ray, be worth less reimbursement, than treating pneumonia without performing the radiograph?

Because Congress has already authorized Medicare to offer accountable care payments under the PPACA, there are many ACO's popping up around the country. These are new enough that the jury is still out as to the effectiveness of these programs. My experience and deductive reasoning cause me significant hesitance and concern regarding the overall benefit of ACO's. Unfortunately, like each of our many different attempts to manage health care in America, I suspect this program will follow a similar course of the past programs like the HMO's the PPO's and the DRG's.

As with everything in medicine, no solution is straight forward or simple. Every topic is complex and multi-faceted. None of the problems facing our nation with regards to our health care have easy solutions. The issues are far more complex than we realize. To think that the solution lies within the pages of the PPACA or the ACO is naïve and mis-informed. History shows us that solutions rarely come from Congress. Remember Ronald Reagan's warning of the nine most feared words in the English language, "I'm from the government and I'm here to help." His statement should remind the nation to turn and run the other way as fast and furiously as possible any time Congress even suggests they have the answers.

15

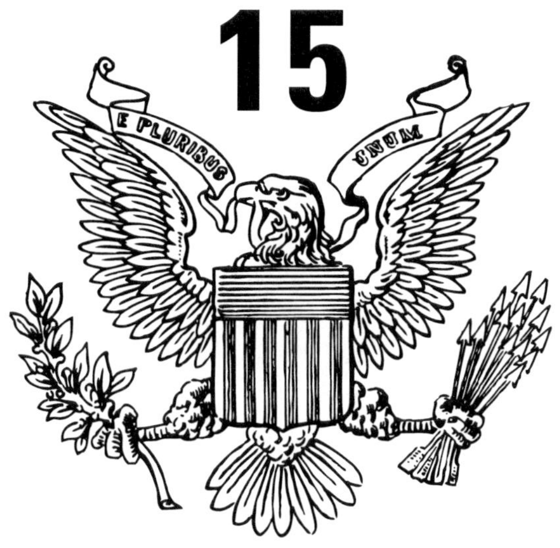

IPAB

Have you heard of the Independent Payment Advisory Board (IPAB)? There are 159 different boards that already have been or will be formed because of the health reform bill. Most of these boards are branches under the HHS, and each one has an appointed board of directors. The purpose, roles, and responsibilities of each of the 159 boards are defined in the PPACA legislation.[1]

The IPAB is a panel of fifteen bureaucrats who are appointed to the IPAB with the sole responsibility of making Medicare cuts. The IPAB is responsible for cutting current Medicare spending by 0.5 percent in 2014, 1.0 percent in 2015, and 1.5 percent in 2016.[2]

To achieve these spending cuts, the IPAB currently intends to reduce the rates that Medicare pays for medical procedures and drugs. Those expenditures that are deemed inefficient (as reported by the comparative-effectiveness research board—one of the other 159 boards created by the PPACA) could be denied altogether. But the current administration and the congressional supporters of the

PPACA remind us that the language in the PPACA specifically prohibits rationing of care. Call it whatever you like, but whenever the IPAB reduces rates for medical procedures and for drugs or denies coverage of a medical service or a medication under the appearance of cost containment, the direct repercussions of cost containment are rationing or limiting care. This is how the PPACA gets around the idea of rationing of medical care; they call it "controlling costs" or "cost containment."

Surveys show that many doctors already limit the number of Medicare patients they see because the rates are too low.[3] Further cuts will have the same effect as when fewer doctors chose to participate in Medicaid; seniors will not be able to find a doctor who is accepting Medicare patients. Also, certain procedures have already been targeted for deep cuts because our bureaucrats have determined them unnecessary. These bureaucrats now know more about medicine than the actual doctors. This is what happens when politicians play doctor; they ultimately ration care.

The IPAB has constitutional problems, too. When the IPAB issues their recommendations for Medicare spending cuts, Congress has the authority to change the IPAB recommendations and enact their own plan, as long as they cut the required percentage. The Senate has the power to override the IPAB decisions with a three-fifths majority vote. However, if the Senate's vote fails, the IPAB recommendations then become law without involvement of any elected officials.[4] If that's not concerning enough, the law forbids judicial review of the IPAB recommendations and fails to explain the process for which a future Congress can discontinue the IPAB.

Does this mean that this board can make some pretty serious decisions regarding medical treatment? What if your eighty-five-year-old mother needs open heart surgery? What if she isn't your ordinary eighty-five-year-old woman but is healthier than many sixty-five-year-olds? What if her family medical history suggests that she's actually a pretty good candidate for this surgery because both of her parents lived well into their nineties? But the surgery costs Medicare a total (on average) of $38,000. Will the IPAB be making these types of decisions, or will the decisions be up to the patient, doctors, and family members? Under these circumstances, I can see how the name "death panel" came about.[5] Isn't that exactly what this panel is?

If America really understood the serious problems that a board like the IPAB can cause, it would be surprising if this panel were even a part of the legislation. But don't forget Nancy Pelosi's famous statement: "[W]e have to pass this bill so that you can find out what is in it." She wasn't kidding!

A Harvard study was performed in 2007 to specifically take a look at the employer mandate requiring that businesses provide health insurance for their employees.[6] This study looked at three possible options for the uninsured to gain health insurance: through the employer mandate, through expansion of Medicaid to 300 percent the federal poverty guideline, and by granting the employer tax credits. Here are the results: Although the employer mandate may result in the greatest decrease in the number of uninsured people, it does so at the highest cost of these three options in terms of lost jobs, forgone wages, and increased employer spending. A Medicaid expansion will actually increase insurance at nearly the same rate as the employer mandate. And tax credits had the least effect on increasing the number of insured people.

Therefore, if the employer mandate has this much of a negative effect on the employer, how many employers will comply with this mandate? Many would probably accept the fine and encourage their employees to turn to the exchanges for their insurance needs, or they may cut their number of full-time and actual employees and turn to part-time workers and agency or outsourced services for their needs. Also, the study clearly showed that adding a mandate for health insurance to the employer's responsibilities would translate into a decrease in wages. The employees may get health insurance—but at what cost to them? Ultimately, the cost is a pay cut.

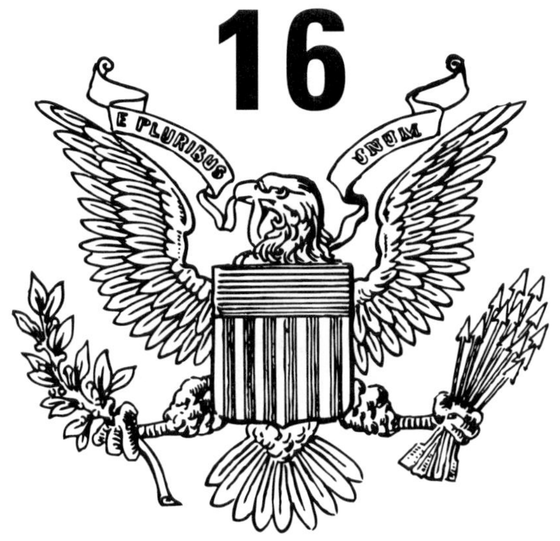

16

HOW DID THIS HAPPEN?

"**A**fter a century of striving, after a year of debate, after a historic vote, health care reform is no longer an unmet promise. It is the law of the land."

—President Barack Obama

President Obama signed the PPACA into law on Tuesday, March 23, 2010.[1] The Democrat obsession with nationalized health care began with Franklin Delano Roosevelt in the 1930s. About eighty years later, through multiple failed attempts and slow, methodical "baby steps" of forcing the government into our doctors' waiting and examination rooms, into our surgeons' operating rooms, and into our cardiologists' procedure rooms, the government has finally succeeded in forcing themselves into every crack and crevice of the American health care system. As President Obama stated clearly, this PPACA is now the law of the land.

Did America really agree? Did its citizens really want this? A national NBC/*Wall Street Journal* poll on January 19, 2010, found that only 33 percent of the American people thought the health reform bill was a good idea, whereas 46 percent thought it was a bad idea.[2] That means 21 percent were undecided. Let's attempt a logical, reasonable, hypothetical exercise to look closely at these numbers. Of those 21 percent, even under the best persuasive rhetoric circumstances, there's no way that all these "undecideds" could have been convinced that health care reform was a good idea. Using an extremely conservative hypothetical argument, if only 4 percent of the 21 percent decided health reform was a bad idea, then even after the most aggressive media campaign to try to convince public opinion, the country would be split at 50:50, for and against—definitely not a public mandate to force health reform on the American people. A more realistic number would be to take the 21 percent of undecided's, throw the talking points for and against the health reform bill at them, and insist on a decision. A more realistic breakdown of the total would be a split right down the middle into 10.5 percent for health reform and 10.5 percent against it. Continuing this hypothetical discussion of these poll numbers, that would clearly make our statistics as 56.5 percent against health reform and 42.5 percent for it.

It seems clear to me that America did not want this legislation. Remember, this poll was in January, two months before the bill was signed, and was taken after the current administration and all the supporters of the PPACA had been on the health reform public awareness tour for at least the previous ten months. After ten months of solid propaganda to try to convince our society, they still convinced only 33 percent of Americans that health reform was a good idea.

Another poll was conducted by CNN from March 19 to 20, 2010, just days before the final congressional vote and passage of the PPACA. This poll found that 59 percent of Americans clearly opposed the bill. After two more months of persuasive and informative tactics, only 39 percent were in favor of it.[3] Rasmussen Reports conducted a poll just before the vote and showed that 54 percent of Americans opposed the bill and 41 percent supported it. Just after its passage, 50 percent of Americans opposed the bill and 46 percent supported it.[4]

Why did Congress pass this legislation? If, around every turn, the politicians were given clear and concise opinions from the American people, then why did they insist on the passage of something that America did NOT want? I'll tell you why. First, they believe that they know more than you. They are better than you at determining what is good for you. Another way to look at this is that, despite you and your limited ability to know what is best for you, they must make these tough decisions for you, and some day you'll see how wise they were. Another reason is their unwavering obsession with health reform. The Democrats' tenacity with this issue was amazing. What other group of people would hang on to a specific issue for nearly eighty years? That's what the Democrats did; they refused to take their eye off the ball until they finally crossed the goal line. Their determination was impressive. Why can't they use this same determination to cut spending and to reduce the deficit? That's because of the third reason they insisted on health reform: They like government. They believe that government is the answer. Most of them really are more socialistic than democratic.

When Ronald Reagan said the nine most dreaded words are "I'm from the government and I'm here to help," he believed it.[5] He understood that what made America great was its limited role of government. When America is at its greatest, the government is not involved. The truly special and unique qualities of our country—our freedoms, our Capitalism, our private sector, our entrepreneurialism, and the exceptionalism of America's citizens—are what make America the greatest country ever!

I've described most of the details in the PPACA, and I've given my opinion where I think the bill is flat out wrong and how implementing these specific parts of the bill would be disastrous for you the patient, me the physician, and the system as a whole. I've also discussed a couple of things that we should consider to make our system better, like tort reform. Now, I'd like to take a look at some ways to improve our current system. These are things that must be improved if we are to repeal the PPACA and begin to correct the problems we face regarding health care and specifically health insurance.

The PPACA can be repealed. On May 22 and 23, 2011, a Rasmussen Reports poll of 1,000 likely voters revealed that 63 percent want the health reform bill, the PPACA, repealed in its entirety.[6] That sounds like a majority. It also sounds like a mandate. Then let's get to it and get it repealed.

Let's pretend that America woke up tomorrow, made all kinds of noise, and managed to persuade Congress to scrap the PPACA. If that would ever happen (and it really could if those of us who are against it—and the polls suggest that this number is a significant majority—would use the same tenacity to get the PPACA repealed that the Democrats used over the course of nearly eighty years to accomplish nationalized health care), then it would be imperative that we solve the many issues that are currently driving up costs in health care. I hope I have convinced you that we actually do receive the best health care in the world right here in America. If this premise is true, then we need only to focus on the costs side and the health insurance side of health care, for the delivery of health care is working well (with perhaps only a couple of exceptions).

I entered medical school in August of 1986 in Kansas City. I've been engulfed in the delivery of medicine since that time, including providing care in two different specialties, family medicine and diagnostic radiology, and one subspecialty, interventional radiology. As a participant in health care, and because of my training in various parts of the country (Kansas City [Kansas and Missouri]; Palm Beach, Florida; Tulsa, Oklahoma; Denver, Colorado; Washington, DC; and rural Missouri and Kansas), I have observed many different health delivery models, and all are working. I have also participated in the health insurance system from a physician or provider perspective. These experiences have allowed me a unique observational and active participant role that has provided me invaluable insight about the problems with our current health care system and about some real and doable solutions. The premise behind my solutions is that there must first be a recognition that many of the problems we currently face were created by government policies and regulations that caused a large divide between three groups of people: the insurance carriers (the patients), the insurance providers (physicians, health professionals, health care services, and hospitals), and the insurance industry (health insurance companies and public health programs like the CMS [Medicare and Medicaid]). To solve these problems, we need less government involvement and more private sector solutions. According to the CMS, by 2019, the government will be responsible for 52 percent of America's health care spending.[7] That means 52¢ of every dollar spent on health care will go toward paying for a government health program. The level of bureaucracy and the number of government employees that the government will bring to health care will only drive the health care costs higher and higher. That's what happens when our government gets involved, and that's what President Obama wants. In 2008, he said, "Under the plan, if you like your current health insurance, nothing changes, except your costs will go down."[8] I hope I've been successful in proving to you that your costs will not go down; they will actually go up. I also hope I have been successful in convincing you that your current health insurance (if you do happen to like it) will actually change significantly under the PPACA. It will probably limit many of the services you already have available. This rationing of care will happen under the disguise of cost containment.

These are the real changes that our current health insurance system needs. The number-one solution that will bring an instant decrease in overall insurance and health care expenses is tort reform.

As I described in chapter 3, 73 percent of doctors in a nationwide Gallup poll said that they practiced defensive medicine. Jackson Healthcare estimates that $650 billion of the $2.5 trillion spent on health care last year in 2010 went to unnecessary diagnostic studies and tests to prevent doctors from being sued for medical malpractice.[9] When Texas implemented medical tort reform in late 2010, they saw a significant decrease in health care costs.[10] But what about the legitimate negligence? There is some legitimate negligence, but it is nowhere near the level that the current legal system claims. I have been through two medical liability lawsuits in twenty-four years. Every doctor now realizes that it's not a matter of if they get sued during their career but when. That's a sad commentary on our legal system and our "someone must be to blame" societal attitude. Both of my cases should never have gone to trial. One was a reaction to a medication, which was settled right before the trial for payment of medical bills incurred during this allergic reaction.

The second one was absolutely frivolous. A patient died, and a wrongful-death suit for medical negligence was filed against me and the hospital where I was covering the emergency department as an FP. On a Saturday afternoon, the patient had presented with chest pain to a hospital emergency department in rural Oklahoma. An expensive but appropriate workup was performed to prove that this man was not having a heart attack. After eight hours of lab tests and workup, the studies showed that his heart was not experiencing a lack of oxygen; he did not have a heart attack. I sent the patient home on Sunday morning with some antibiotics for a possible lung infection and with strict instructions to follow up with his doctor on Monday morning. Because we were in a small town, I was even able to arrange his appointment with his PCP for 9:00 am Monday. The patient did not keep his appointment. He went to work on Monday and Tuesday. He did not go to work on Wednesday. On Thursday, he was found deceased in his apartment. It appeared that he had been drinking alcohol in excess, for several beer bottles were found next to him; however, the probability of him having been drinking was not admissible in court. He apparently died of a pulmonary embolus (a clot to the vessels in his lungs), but he had not shown any signs of a clot in his legs. The cause of death was not confirmed at autopsy. The family sued me and the hospital for wrongful death and medical negligence.

I was in radiology residency at the time of this case and had been covering an emergency department in a small town to make a little extra money (medical residents make right at the federal poverty guideline).[11] The case took more than three years to go to trial. By the time it went to trial, I had completed my residency training and my fellowship and was now practicing radiology in Topeka, Kansas. I spent tens of hours driving from Kansas to Oklahoma for depositions. The stress of this case caused my family and me much anguish. Few people really can understand what it's like for a doctor to lose a patient—any patient—especially when the doctor did everything he knew to treat the patient appropriately. The case ultimately went to jury trial. Medical malpractice cases go to a jury trial in almost every state. The jury was composed of people from this small town. I was considered an outsider. The highest level of education on the jury was completion of the twelfth grade, which did not make this jury a jury of my peers. The plaintiff's lawyer was an attorney who lived in the small town. The plaintiff's expert witness was a doctor who hadn't practiced medicine in twenty-five years. He had practiced emergency medicine early in his career but had begun doing medical malpractice cases as an expert witness. This had grown into a profession for him, and he left the practice of medicine. He was a polished and well-spoken man who did legal work for a living. He also made about $3,500 for each trial. During one of the trial's breaks, he told me he participated in anywhere from 180 to 200 trials a year. (This comes to nearly $665,000 a year, three times more than I had ever made as a doctor practicing medicine.) This doctor—the expert witness—made me and my diagnostic skills look inept. By the time the trial was over, I wondered how I had even managed to pass my boards in three different specialties.

The plaintiff won the case. Because I was a resident and didn't have a great malpractice policy, I was dropped from the case right before the verdict was read, and the plaintiff sued only the local hospital. The jury awarded the plaintiff $2.5 million. Had I not been dropped from the case, I probably couldn't have had another malpractice insurance carrier to ever cover me again, and I might have never practiced medicine again. To this day, I still do not know what this patient really died of. I have studied this case hundreds of times over the years, trying to see what I did incorrectly (if anything) and how I could have saved this patient. After fifteen years, I still don't know what I would have done better. Sometimes, people die. Sometimes, we can't save them. That doesn't mean I don't and that I haven't made mistakes in medicine, for I have. But with this case, I don't know what my mistakes were, if I made any at all.

I determined that the entire trial was a theatrical performance. The plaintiff's expert witness was a polished and persuasive actor who convinced the jury that I was a poorly educated hack who should not have been practicing emergency medicine. At one point in the trial, he even stated that I probably got out of family medicine and went to radiology because I actually realized that I wasn't very good at patient care. This was from a man who hadn't seen a patient in twenty-five years. The plaintiff paid $3,500 for this professional hired gun who had the experience to make me look really inept, and he succeeded royally. In my profession, we refer to these paid professionals as prostitutes.

When we talk of health care reform and we don't even consider tort reform, you can see why this issue is very personal to me. Because of this one particular case, I know without a doubt that I practice defensive medicine. When I hear other doctors admit that they do, too, I do NOT blame them or look at them with disdain. Practicing defensive medicine is what doctors do in this medico-legal environment; they order extra tests, no matter what the cost, to take care of the patient and to keep from being sued. If I could be critical of how I handled this case at all, I've often wondered why I didn't just order a CT scan and be done with it. But I was practicing cost-effective medicine. Yet I remind myself that a pulmonary embolus won't show up on a CT scan unless it is occurring at the time of the scan, and the patient is always short of breathe with such a blockage. This man, however, was not.

What about the legitimate negligence? The plaintiff was convinced I was negligent and that they had a shot at winning this case. Should they have been allowed to take this to trial? I believe that a better system would be to have a state medico-legal board of health professionals and laypeople appointed by each state governor. The board's role would be to first study each individual claim of medical negligence and then decide if the case were frivolous or if negligence had occurred. Frivolous cases would be thrown out, whereas the others would then go to trial. Some states have a system like this already in place. I also believe that there should be a cap on the amount of money that can be awarded for negligence. Medical tort would absolutely decrease much of the cost of health care, both from an insurance side and from a delivery side. We must have medical tort reform to improve our current health system. It's time to stand up to the American Association for Justice and demand that we improve this system.

Let's look at another problem and a plausible solution. Does the government buy your car insurance? How about your homeowner's policy? What about disability and life insurance? What about employers? Do they buy these insurance policies for their workers? No, as a rule, they don't. Then why should they buy your health insurance? During World War II, employers began to provide health insurance for their workers because the US government imposed wage controls and salary freezes. That's correct; the government said our nation was at war and needed all the money to win the war, so employers were prohibited from granting their employees wage increases during this difficult time in America's history. To give their loyal workers something, employers decided to pay for their health insurance. In case you didn't know it, World War II ended in 1945. So, why didn't employer-sponsored health insurance coverage end back then, too? Often, once programs and ideas are implemented (especially taxes), they're nearly impossible to shake. When employees are not paying directly for their health insurance, they don't realize the overall expenses, and they don't attempt to locate less-expensive health policies. But when workers do buy their own insurance, they tend to shop around for the best policy for their needs; therefore, because of competition, the insurance costs come down. Instead of demanding an employer mandate to provide insurance for all its employees, we need just the opposite: Get the employers out of the business of providing health insurance for their workers. Americans like choice. We want to make choices for everything we purchase. This is how we develop a flexible and innovative health insurance industry. All citizens—not their employers—should own their own health insurance policy.

Similarly, each personally owned insurance policy must be portable. If you change jobs, you should be allowed to take your health insurance policy with you. Rather than employers managing your health insurance policy, you should manage your own policy. If you return to school, you should manage your own policy. If you take personal time off or personal leave, you should manage your own policy. I know this is a change from what many Americans are used to, but this is what you do with your car or your homeowners insurance, isn't it? Employees would no longer feel trapped in a job they didn't like or want because of their health benefits. This would also allow for competition in the health insurance industry, just like the automotive and homeowners insurance industries.

If you want to buy a car, are you required to buy it in your state? You may choose to shop locally for convenience, but there are no government requirements that say you can't purchase your car in any other state than the one you live in. So, why isn't health insurance this way? It's because of all the state mandates or regulations. It gets too confusing for insurances to meet the requirements of all fifty states. We should do away with the state mandates or make them all the same and allow consumers to purchase the best health insurance policy for their needs, regardless of which state they buy this policy from. If Congress were interested in real health care reform, they would tear down the state limitation walls and open up the marketplace for real reform. Instead, they throw 2,562 pages of obstructive and intrusive legislation at us without even addressing this well-known and impeding problem.

Regarding your car insurance, when you pull up to the gas pump, do you expect your insurance policy to cover the gasoline to fill up your car? Of course you don't. That's not the reason that insurance was developed from the beginning. Insurance was originally designed to be a "safety net" to provide you and your family with security in the event of a catastrophe. Any form of insurance, whether automotive, homeowners, or even health, was initially designed to provide coverage or security in the event of a major accident, like a car accident, if your home burned down, or if you developed a catastrophic medical illness. If we would return insurance coverage to its intended purpose, and if we would put the other day-to-day routine medical costs back into the consumer's hands, the cost of medicine would come down.

The private sector works. When competition is encouraged, prices come down. An excellent example of this is cosmetic, elective breast augmentation surgery. In the past decade, when all other costs in medicine have increased, the price for breast augmentation surgery has decreased. Why? Because the private sector and competition works. When an elective procedure is not covered by your insurance policy, and really elective cosmetic procedures should not be covered by insurance policies as this goes against the real purpose for insurance, then the patient becomes a consumer. As a consumer they search for the best prices for their medical treatment or medical procedure. Under these circumstances, the consumer keeps the supplier (the surgeon) honest and fair minded, thus preventing the costs from arbitrarily going up at the doctor's whim, the insurance company's greed, or the government's incompetence. When we return insurance to its intended purpose, and when we allow the American people to again be consumers of their own health care, we will see the prices dramatically decrease and ultimately stabilize to a reasonable and realistic fee schedule.

One of the best ways to incentivize the American people is to allow them to use tax-free dollars for their health insurance and health care. Plenty of Americans want to save their own money to pay for their own medical care. These are the folks who follow the Dave Ramsey financial planning model,[12] who emulate the *Millionaire Next Door* model,[13] or who are just plain ordinary folks who refuse to let anyone else (including our government) pay their own way. These responsible, proactive, and frugal citizens believe that it's their personal responsibility to pay their own way in any and all aspects of their lives, including their health care. These Americans should be respected, imitated, and even rewarded for their conscientious behavior. Why not allow these responsible people to use tax-free dollars for their medical care? An exceptional vehicle to accomplish tax-free savings is the already available health savings account (HSA).[14] These accounts were designed to encourage people to manage their own money carefully and to take an active role in their health care. These HSAs work. They encourage competition among health care providers, and these providers therefore compete for you as their client, just as any merchant strives to gain your loyalty and your business. Generally speaking, the providers actually like this approach. Once they have earned your business and you have chosen to see them for your health care, they can actually be paid cash for their services—a novel idea!

And you, the consumer, generally like this approach because you are treated like a valued customer. The providers look at you as a customer who can go anywhere you choose for your health care, so they do the little extra things to meet your needs. They also realize that if they do not serve you in a professional and attentive manner, you can move on down the road to the next doctor's office. This competition actually enhances your experience with your doctor and improves overall satisfaction.

America already understands the value of the HSA. Currently, 10 million Americans have HSA-eligible accounts,[15] according to America's Health Insurance Plans, a national association for health insurance companies. Unfortunately, Congress is looking at ways to cut HSAs and limit or eliminate pretax programs altogether. In 2011, the HSA can no longer be used for over-the-counter medication.[16] Anyone making a nonmedical withdrawal from his or her account will face higher penalties. That's what happens when the members of Congress like big government; they obstruct the free market. If we are serious about cutting health care costs, we need to turn to HSAs, FSAs, health reimbursement accounts, and Archer medical savings accounts as some tax-free ways for responsible individuals to participate in managing the costs of their health care.

We must do away with all these state mandates. Quit telling insurance companies that they must accept anyone regardless of preexisting conditions. Instead, require that the insurance companies offer a variety of plans that meet different needs for the various types of circumstances. We know that a one-size-fits-all approach doesn't work. If the mandates are removed the insurance companies have suggested they will offer more variety of heal insurance plans.

If you entered any major tertiary care facility and walked into the intensive care unit (ICU), you would likely find at least three people with a similar disease process laying in adjacent hospital beds. Let's say you entered the neurological ICU and in three beds there were three different patients who had recently suffered a stroke. Let's say each patient was in their early sixties and they each had a different form of health insurance coverage. For this realistic example let's say that one patient has already qualified for Medicare coverage, the second patient has Medicaid coverage, and the third patient has private health insurance from a reputable and well known insurance company. We'll also assume that all three patients suffered their stroke on the same day, and that they entered the ICU within hours of each other. And for the sake of discussion, let's suggest that they are receiving basically the same medical treatment. Here's what most American's don't realize, each of these patients will be charged a completely different price for essentially the same disease state and treatment. That's correct, three different forms of health coverage, and three different fee schedules for the same disease and treatment. Are you surprised? If three different people went to the grocery store and they all purchased the same items, should they expect to pay the same price? Most thoughtful people would answer a definitive "yes"! In American medicine, that's not the case.

The reason that there are three different costs associated with the same disease and treatment is because the government, even though they have gone about regulating every other aspect of health care, is convinced that they know what's best for each of us, and therefore they should be able to determine what they will reimburse doctors and hospitals for their Medicare and Medicaid patients. However, to try and maintain control, they have allowed hospitals and doctors to charge more to private insurance patients for similar medical treatment, in order to make up for the continually decreasing reimbursement from Medicare and Medicaid. The government has basically said doctors shouldn't complain about the continual, yearly cuts in Medicare and Medicaid reimbursements, instead, they should simply make up the difference by charging more to the private insurance companies. After all, they're part of the wealthy and evil insurance industry, so they can afford, and should even be required to pay more, just because they are members of the "haves" segment of society. If the government throws us a bone, we might not be as quick to draw attention to the disparity or inequity built into the current system.

We need transparency in medicine. Hospitals and doctors should be willing to show any patient what they're expected cost for any medical service will be. This could be in the form of an estimate, no different than a contractor who comes to remodel your home provides you with a quote for the cost to complete your project. A patient could get three estimates or quotes from three different doctors, just as they would if they were remodeling their bathroom, and then choose accordingly based on price, quality, testimony, and previous outcome. Each doctor should be allowed to set their own fee schedules, rather than be forced to accept the fee schedules forced on each physician by Medicare. And each patient should be able to reasonably shop for the best price, as they do in all other walks of life. This puts the cost containment back into the consumer's hands, rather in the insurance company's or the federal government's hands. And for the true emergency, insurance would serve its intended purpose, and cover the emergency or catastrophic medical fees.

With an inevitable shortage of doctors, this problem needs some real solutions. Encourage college students to go into medicine. Give tax deductions for student loans, including medical education loans. Set up a more-attractive program that encourages medical students to go into a primary care area of medicine, including such things as a loan-repayment program based on years of service in underserved counties across the world. Increase the salaries of FPs and pediatricians so that family doctors' incomes are more in line with the specialists' incomes. This could happen in the form of significant increases in Medicare payment to FPs. The 10 percent increase will do little to attract students to family medicine, so make it a real increase of 50 percent or more. Finally, reward doctors with increased pay if they oversee PAs. This would allow each doctor to oversee anywhere from five to ten NPs or PAs, enabling him to be the "captain of the ship" and available for any questions the NPs or PAs may have. The FP could deal with the cases with higher-level acuity and the hospitalized patients. This would allow PCPs and primary care practices to see many more patients and to function more efficiently. We may face a current physician shortage in America, but there are some real solutions if we begin thoughtful planning and methodical implementation now.

For years now, vouchers have been proposed for private schooling in America, but this has continued to fall on deaf ears. Vouchers could be extremely effective in health care, too. Why not give the poor citizens a voucher that is good for $3,600 worth of health insurance premiums? The individuals, if they qualified, could purchase a health insurance policy of their choice. This would be easy to implement. There would not need to be a massive and expensive agency to put the voucher system in motion. All that would be needed is a small staff who process the applications, oversee the program for fraud and abuse, and send out the vouchers to the qualified applicants. This is much easier than the current proposals for the poor in the PPACA. I suspect that this solution is not complex enough to get Washington's attention, yes?

I think one of the best ways that we, as a country, can recover much of our lost revenue could be done in one simple step: Freeze the current congressional salaries. It has always amazed and irritated me at the same time that when the rest of the country is cinching up their belts in a down economy, and when most workers and small businesses are lucky to maintain their current salaries without any wage increases (and keeping up with cost of living or inflationary increases), our Congress has no qualms at all about voting themselves at least cost-of-living salary increases. I think Congress should never be allowed to vote themselves a salary increase. (Apparently, they won't call their salary increase what it is: an increase in their pay. Instead, they use the term "COLA," or cost of living adjustment. This COLA is set at 3 percent and automatically occurs without their vote, unless they purposefully elect to vote the COLA down.)[17] Congress says that all they did with their salaries was maintain their COLA. Why not freeze their current salary for the next five years? How much revenue would that generate? It would definitely generate several million dollars' worth of savings. More importantly, it would go a long way with gaining respect and appreciation from the American people. Or, why not base any change in salary on Congress's ability to balance the budget? Or, better yet, if Congress would actually come in under budget, then they could have their COLA wage increases.

Unfortunately, a $1 million savings today for Congress almost seems insignificant or of no benefit, so why even worry about this little amount? Wouldn't it be nice to have that problem, having complete and unlimited access to other people's money for your own salary increases? What a problem to have. If we implemented term limits, no longer would going to Washington be a career. The system was never designed to have career politicians, and yet that's exactly what most of them have become. Career politicians couldn't exist with term limits, and their COLA would not be too important to them. Or, perhaps we decide that going to Congress for a term limit should be a charitable act. Each congressperson could donate his or her time. We could implement no pay for politicians for three or five years, or we could pay them the going rate of a soldier or a military serviceperson who is serving our country. It would be interesting to see just how much money the country would save. This would undoubtedly change Congress's perspective for a while. And while we are discussing a congressional salary freeze, why not lower taxes for all of America? It has been proved time and again that a tax cut stimulates our economy. People have more discretionary income, and generally Americans are more than willing to spend this right back into the American economy. Or, if a tax cut isn't your thing, then why not reform the IRS and Title 26? Many studies support that a consumption tax, national sales tax, or flat tax in place of our current federal income tax would generate more revenue in taxes than our current system. Cutting or eliminating the bloated bureaucracy of the IRS would generate significant savings. This would be another practical and simple way to raise money that could be put into Medicare and Medicare reimbursements.

Of course, it is clear that I would like to see the PPACA repealed. In my opinion, that would be the best initial action that we could do as a country so we could then begin down the path of real reform. However, if the PPACA is not repealed and that it is here to stay, then ALL exemptions must be eliminated. All Americans should be required to participate. Why on earth should Muslims and Native Americans be exempt from this bill? Why should anyone be exempt because of their religious beliefs? If there were any logic in religious exemptions, then I would like to claim right here and now that it is against my religious belief and convictions to pay taxes. I am already tithing 10 percent of my income to God. Why must I give another 38 percent to the government? If all blessings (including money) come from God, then it is against my religious beliefs to pay taxes or tithes to anyone other than God. Therefore, I am formally requesting my exemption from the federal tax system; while I'm at it, I'd like to just go ahead and get that PPACA exemption for my Christian beliefs as well. (Didn't I tell you I'm a Christian Scientist? All doctors who believe in Christianity are.) Of course, I cannot see any logical reason why Muslims or illegal immigrants should ever be exempt from the PPACA. If we refuse to deport the illegal immigrants, we should at least make them pay more than their fair share. (If I were illegally in any country, no other society would even consider letting me stay, and to provide me health insurance would be unheard of!) Remind me why Muslims are exempt again. The most egregious exemption of all is our own Congress. This PPACA health reform legislation isn't good enough for them, but it is for the rest of us. If you can't see any other reason why the PPACA is a bad idea, this one fact should convince you. Congress should not be exempt from any of their legislation—ever. That should be our benchmark with all legislation. If Congress agrees to participate, then we should take a serious look at the bill; however, if they exempt themselves, the bill should automatically be thrown out.

Finally, doctors should be able to receive a tax deduction for any charitable care they currently give. If doctors were allowed to deduct from their taxes the number of hours they saw the uninsured and indigent patients in our society, and then if they were to multiply this figure by their current hourly rate, they would have a real and significant reason to donate their time and talents to assist the impoverished. This would also help with the physician shortage because many of the doctors who are retired or semiretired might be more willing to donate their time if they actually saw some small benefit to them, too. I'm sure that Congress wouldn't even consider this because they perceive doctors as already making way too much money; can't the doctors just donate their time without any benefit to them? Isn't that why it's called a donation? Actually, if anyone else makes any other type of charitable donation to the poor, don't they get to deduct that from their taxes? If a Little League team needs bats and helmets and the local sporting goods store donates these items, doesn't the store get to deduct the value of these items from their taxes? If the doctor's product is his time and expertise, then he should also be allowed to deduct the fair market value for his time.

Each of these solutions is better than the PPACA. It is time for us to consider some true reform that limits the far-reaching and intrusive power of government and places health insurance and health care back in the hands of the private sector. It's only through these types of simple and practical solutions that we can once again make the practice of medicine the enjoyable and attractive profession that it used to be. This is my father's health profession. Maybe it's time we returned to the tried-and-true principles that made this country great: less government, more free-market competition, tax benefits, and incentives for patients and providers to find the most affordable plans and practices. If we would turn to the solutions I listed instead of the PPACA, I believe that we would restore the public's confidence in the health profession and restore the providers' trust that the system is there to assist them in offering the best health care to their patients.

The newly elected Congress in 2010 based their election promises on a platform of repeal of the PPACA. The changes in Congress were significant in the possibility for actual repeal; the momentum the opposition to the PPACA gained must be continued. If a new president is elected in 2012 (and that could be a real possibility if the contender keeps an eye on the repeal of the PPACA and makes it a major plank in his or her platform), then repeal not only would be a possibility but also would actually stand a good chance of becoming a reality. Don't let up on your continual push to repeal the PPACA. We must maintain a steady drumbeat to get to the goal line. Pretend we are at the fifty-yard line and we have to get to the end zone by November 2012. To do this, we will need to chew up some clock, keep the ball on the ground, not make any mistakes, and push the health reform team back with each play. This can be done. But it won't be easy.

America remains the freest country with the greatest wealth in the history of civilization. The socialist agenda over the past ninety years has slowly eroded the firm foundation of our republic. This foundation can be repaired, and repealing the PPACA is a giant step toward this goal. Don't be duped when you hear the words "I'm from the government and I'm here to help." Instead, run the other direction as fast as you can. Whenever someone from government comes to the rescue, it always ends up costing someone else a whole lot of money.

The American system of democracy is one of the most sophisticated systems in history. I have an unwavering support for our government and our republic; however, I have lost complete trust in the individuals who occupy the various seats of Congress. It appears that no one is listening. Americans spoke, and they did not want this particular health care reform legislation, but the members of Congress forced their will on them. However, because we do have the freedoms and privileges as Americans citizens, we do have the right to free speech, and I can voice my own opinion as I have throughout much of this book. Therefore, I can attempt to convince you that the PPACA must be repealed, but I suspect many of you already know that. For those of you who support this piece of legislation, I'd be more than happy to let you have it. Perhaps I could opt out?

Our founding fathers understood that each individual American citizen has the right to life, liberty, and the pursuit of happiness.[18] Health care is not a right but a privilege that comes with a price tag. Don't let the PPACA and our socialist-leaning Congress take away your liberties. All these freedoms—the freedom to choose your physician, the freedom to choose the best health plan for you and your family, and the freedom to decide the fate of your medical care—are your rights as Americans.

BIBLIOGRAPHY

CHAPTER 1

1   "Nancy Pelosi: We have to pass the bill so that you can find out what is in it," BuzzFlash, March 22, 2010; available at: http://blog.buzzflash.com/alerts/810

2   ARC Press Release, "Nancy Pelosi vs. the Founding Fathers," Ayn Rand Center, March 24, 2010; available at: http://www.solopassion.com/node/7500

3   Office of the Speaker of the House, "Pelosi Remarks at the 2010 Legislative Conference for National Association of Counties," PR Newswire, March 9, 2010; available at: http://www.prnewswire.com/news-releases/ 87131117.html

4   USA Statistics, U.S. Census Bureau, June 3, 2011; available at: http://quickfacts.census.gov/qfd/states/00000.html

5   Reports and Studies, "The Report to the President of the Committee on Economic Security," Social Security Agency, http://www.ssa.gov/history/reports/ces.html, {accessed July 16th, 2011}

6   Kimberly Lankford, "The Social Security Debate," Kiplinger, March 17,2005; available at: http://www.kiplinger.com/features/archives/2005/03/ssprimer.html

7   Social Security Agency, "Organizational History of SSA," available at: http://www.ssa.gov/history/orghist.html, {accessed June 25th, 2011}

8   John Woolley and Gerhard Peters, "The American Presidency Project: Franklin D Roosevelt 17-Message to Congress on the National Health Program," January 23, 1939; available at: http://www.presidency.ucsb.edu/ws/index.php?pid=15699#axzz1Sxb16FWO

9   Karen S. Palmer, "A Brief History: Universal Health Care Efforts in the US," PNHP, Physician's for a National Health Program, Spring, 1999; available at: http://www.pnhp.org/facts/a_brief_history_universal_health_care_efforts_in_the_us.php?page=2

10 "Gallup and Fortune Polls, 1940's" Public Opinion Quarterly (1942) 6 (4):650-665, available at: http://poq.oxfordjournals.org/content/6/4/650.abstract

11 Monte M. Poen, "This Day in Truman History November 19, 1945 President Truman's Proposed Health Program," Harry S. Truman Library and Museum, November 19, 1945; available at: http://www.trumanlibrary.org/anniversaries/healthprogram.htm

12 Steve Hoenisch, "Health Care Policy of the Democratic Party," The Encyclopedia of the American Democratic and Republican Parties," July 23rd, 2004; available at: http://www.criticism.com/policy/democrats-health-care-policy.php

13 Social Security History, "Actions in Congress," Social Security Agency, Social Security Amendments, 1956; available at: http://www.socialsecurity.gov/history/tally56.html

14 Social Security History, "Chapter 4: The Fourth Round-1957 to 1965," Social Security Agency, Social Security Amendments, 1960; available at: http://www.socialsecurity.gov/history/tally56.html

15 Thomas J Reid, III, "US Health-Care Reform: Lessons Learned – A brief History of Medicare Legislation and Its Relevance to the Health-Care Reform Debate in the 111th Congress," Digital Journal, September 28, 2009; available at: http://www.digitaljournal.com/blog/4154

16 Charlotte Twight, "Medicare's Origin: The Economics and Politics of Dependency," CATO Journal, 1992; available at: http://www.cato.org/pubs/journal/cj16n3/cj16n3-3.pdf

17 Tom Schatz, "Medicare will be Bankrupt by 2019," The Heartland Institute, May 2004; available at: http://www.heartland.org/policybot/results/14901/Medicare_Will_Be_Bankrupt_by_2019.html

18 "Nancy Pelosi: We have to pass the bill so that you can find out what is in it," BuzzFlash, March 22, 2010; available at: http://blog.buzzflash.com/alerts/810

19 ARC Press Release, "Nancy Pelosi vs. the Founding Fathers," Ayn Rand Center, March 24, 2010; available at: http://www.solopassion.com/node/7500

20 HBMA Government Report, "The Patient Protection and Affordable Act," HBMA Government Office, Spring, 2011; available at: http://www.bilamerica.com/wp-content/uploads/2011/05/Washington Report03042010.pdf

CHAPTER 2

1 "Health Care in the United States," Wikipedia, 2009; available at: http://en.wikipedia.org/wiki/Health_insurance_in_the_United_States

2 Gallup Poll, "About one in six US Adults are without Health Insurance," July 22, 2009; available at: http://www.gallup.com/poll/12820

3 Robert Longley, "Is the US Really That Uninsured?" About.com, US Government Info., 2009; available at: http://usgovinfo.about.com/od/medicarehealthinsurance/a/insurancestats.htm

4 US Census Bureau, "Statistics about Business Size from the US Census Bureau," 2008; available at: http://www.census.gov/econ/smallbus.html

5 Barack Obama, "Health care reform plans being considered in Congress 'will finally reduce the costs of health care,'" Politifact.com, December 15, 2009; available at: http://www.politifact.com/truth-o-meter/statements/2009/dec/18/barack-obama/obama-said-health-care-reform-will-reduce-cost-hea/

6 CBO, "Your unfunded liability for social security Medicare and Medicaid is close to 100 trillion so is there any way to pay these programs without bankrupting America?" Answers.com; available at: http://wiki.answers.com/Q/Your_unfunded_liability_for_Social_Security_Medicare_and_Medicaid_is_close_to_100_trillion_so_is_there_any_way_to_pay_for_these_programs_without_bankrupting_America

7 AHFF Geoff, "CBO: Obamacare = at least $109 Billion in Deficit Spending Over 10 years;" Centrist.net, March 20, 2010, http://centristnetblog.com/daily/cbo-obamacare-at-least-109-billion-in-deficit-spending-over-10-years/

8 US House Budget Committee, "Obamacare: A Budget-Busting, Job-Killing Health Care Law," Report on PPACA from US House Budget

Committee, January 6, 2011; available at: http://www.speaker.gov/UploadedFiles/ObamaCareReport.pdf

9   Mark Schenker, "Former CBO Head Says Deficits to Rise by $562 Billion as Obamacare Not Deficit Neutral," Free Republic, Sunday, March 21,2010; available at: http://www.freerepublic.com/focus/f-bloggers/2475876/posts

10 "US Congress," Wikipedia, 2009; available at: http://en.wikipedia.org/wiki/United_States_Congress

11 "How Long is It? The US Tax Code," Trygve.com, 2006; available at: http://www.trygve.com/taxcode.html

12 HHS Press Office, US Department of Health and Human Services, Tuesday, April 6, 2010; available at: http://www.hhs.gov/news/press/2010pres/04/20100406c.html

13 Dennis Cauchon, "For Feds, More get 6-figure Salaries," USA Today, December, 11,2009; available at: http://www.usatoday.com/news/washington/2009-12-10-federal-pay-salaries_N.htm

14 Mark Kirk, "According to the nonpartisan Congressional Budget Office, the IRS would need to hire over 16,000 people...," Politifact.com, March 21st, 2010: available at: http://www.politifact.com/truth-o-meter/statements/2010/mar/29/mark-kirk/kirk-says-health-care-bill-will-lead-irs-hire-more/

15 Kay Stanley, "Crafting a Sustainable Model for Physician Recruitment and Retention," Coker Group, March, 2009; available at: http://cokergroup.com/files/whitepapers/White_Paper_-_Crafting_a_Sustainable_Model_for_Physician_Recruitment_and_Retention_200904011.pdf

16 "Average Family Practice Physician Salaries," Simply Hired, July 27, 201; available at: http://www.simplyhired.com/a/salary/search/q-family+practice+physician

17 Curtis Copeland, "New Entities Created Pursuant to the Patient Protection and Affordable Care Act," Congressional Research Service, July 8, 2010; available at: http://op.bna.com/mdw.nsf/id/plon-87rjc7/$File/CRSreport.pdf

CHAPTER 3

1   Richard P. Gulla, "Investigation of Defensive Medicine in Massachusetts Study," Massachusetts Medical Society, November 17, 2008; available at: http://www.massmed.org/AM/Template.cfm

2   Gallop Poll, "Physician Study: Quantifying The Cost of Defensive Medicine," Jackson HealthCare, December, 2009; available at: http://www.jacksonhealthcare.com/healthcare-research/healthcare-costs-defensive-medicine-study.aspx

3   Governor Rick Perry, Health Care Reform,ProCon.org, November 1, 2010; available at: http://healthcarereform.procon.org/view.resource.php?resourceID=003725

4   "Top Ten Pros and Cons, Are the March 2010 federal health care reform laws good for America?" November 1, 2010; available at: http://healthcarereform.procon.org/view.resource.php?resourceID=003725

5   Nicholas Ballasy, "Howard Dean: Democrats Left Tort Reform Out of Health Care Bill Because They Feared 'Taking On' Trial Lawyers," CNSNews.com, August 26,2009; available at: http://www.cnsnews.com/node/53126

6   Kevin Mooney, "Trial Lawyers Seek Return on Contributions to Senate Democrats," Beltway Confidential, August 14, 2009; available at: http://washingtonexaminer.com/blogs/beltway-confidential/2009/08/trial-lawyers-seek-return-contributions-senate-democrats

7   David Freddoso, Kevin Mooney, "Trial Lawyers Seek Return on Contributions to Senate Democrats," Washington Examiner, August 14, 2009; available at: http://sroblog.com/2009/08/14/trial-lawyers-seek-return-on-contributions-to-senate-democrats-washington-examiner/http://sroblog.com/2009/08/14/trial-lawyers-seek-return-on-contributions-to-senate-democrats-washington-examiner/

8   Dr. Bob, "Texas Tort Reform," The Doctor Is In, July 26th, 2009; available at: http://docisinblog.com/index.php/2009/07/27/texas-tort-reform/

9   Wilson Elser, "Mississippi Passes Sweeping Tort Reform Bill," Wilson Elser Moskowitz Edelman and Dicker, LLP, June 16, 2004; available at: http://www.wilsonelser.com/Publications/detail.aspx?pub=88

CHAPTER 4

1 CRS Report To Congress, "Summary of Potential Employer Penalties Under PPACA (P.L. 111-148)," Congressional Research Service, April 5, 2010; available at: http://www.ltgov.ri.gov/smallbusiness/employerprovisions.pdf

2 The 2009 HHS Poverty Guidelines, U.S. Department of Health and Human Services; 2009, available at: http://aspe.hhs.gov/poverty/09poverty.shtml

3 Richard S. Foster, "Estimated Financial Effects of the 'Patient Protection and Affordable Care Act,'" Department of Health and Human Services Centers for Medicare and Medicaid, April 22, 2010; available at: http://www.cms.gov/ActuarialStudies/Downloads/PPACA_2010-04-22.pdf

4 Office of the Actuary, "2008 Actuarial Report of the Financial Outlook For Medicaid," Department of Health and Human Services Centers for Medicare and Medicaid, October, 2008; available at: https://www.cms.gov/ActuarialStudies/downloads/MedicaidReport2008.pdf

5 CRS Report To Congress, "Summary of Potential Employer Penalties Under PPACA (P.L. 111-148)," Congressional Research Service, April 5, 2010; available at: http://www.ltgov.ri.gov/smallbusiness/employerprovisions.pdf

6 Michael Tanner, "Bad Medicine, A Guide to the Real Costs and Consequences of the New Health Care Law," The CATO Institute, 2011; available at: http://www.cato.org/pubs/wtpapers/BadMedicineWP.pdf

7 Maggie Mahar, "The Nedicaid Challenge, Part II: Reimbursement and the Federal Government," A Project of the Century Foundation Health Beat, October 9, 2008; available at: http://www.healthbeat-blog.com/2008/10/the-medicaid--1.html

8 "Health Care Reform, Msdicaid and State Budget Woes," State Budget Solutions Real Solutions for Real Budget Problems, March 24, 2010; available at: http://www.statebudgetsolutions.org/publications/detail/health-care-reform-medicaid-and-state-budget-woes

9   "California is Broke-19 Reasons Why it may be Time for Everyone to Leave the State of California for Good," The Economic Collapse, October 22, 2010; available at: http://theeconomiccollapseblog.com/archives/california-is-broke-19-reasons-why-it-may-be-time-for-everyone-to-leave-the-state-of-california-for-good

10 "Fractured-The state of health Care in Texas," The Primary Care Coalition, 2008; available at: http://www.tafp.org/advocacy/fractured.pdf

11 Steven Reinberg, "More Medicaid Patients Using ER's Study Finds," August 10, 2010; available at: http://health.usnews.com/health-news/managing-your-healthcare/insurance/articles/2010/08/10/more-medicaid-patients-using-ers-study-finds

12 "Underpayment by Medicare and Medicaid Fact Sheet," American Hospital Association, November, 2009,; available at: http://www.aha.org/aha/content/2009/pdf/09medicunderpayment.pdf

CHAPTER 5

1   The Free Dictionary, "Mandatory," The Free Dictionary by Farlex, 2010; available at: http://www.thefreedictionary.com/mandatory

2   Independent Association of Businesses, "Half of All States Now Suing to Stop PPACA ," January 14th, 2011; available at: http://iabusa.wordpress.com/2011/01/14/

3   Hadley Heath, "A Severe Mistake for Obama Care," Health Care Lawsuits, November 30, 2010; http://healthcarelawsuits.org/blog/detail.php?c=2390395&t=A-Severe-Mistake-for-ObamaCare

4   Webb Milsaps, Peter Rich, "Supreme Court Receives New Request to Consider Constitutionality of Health Reform Law," July 29, 2011; available at: http://www.healthcarelawreform.com/tags/patient-protection-and-afforda/

5   "Commerce Clause," Cornell Law School, Available at: http://www.law.cornell.edu/wex/commerce_clause

6 Randy E Barnett, "Is Health-care reform constitutional?" The Washington Post, March 21, 2010; available at: http://www.washingtonpost.com/wp-dyn/content/article/2010/03/19/AR2010031901470.html

7 "Are there penalties for not having health insurance?" Health Care Reform, Procon.org, May 26, 2010; available at: http://healthcarereform.procon.org/view.answers.php?questionID=001454

8 "Health Insurance Exemptions," Snopes.com, April 13, 2010; available at: http://www.snopes.com/politics/medical/exemptions.asp

9 "Census Bureau: 46.3 million uninsured in the U.S.'" U.S. Census Bureau, 2008; available at: http://24ahead.com/census-bureau-463-million-uninsured-us-including-95-million-

10 "The Real Uninsured," Fact Check, June 24, 2009; available at: http://www.factcheck.org/2009/06/the-real-uninsured/

11 "The Real Uninsured," Fact Check, June 24, 2009; available at: http://www.factcheck.org/2009/06/the-real-uninsured/

12 Michael Hiltzik, "U.S. Census Bureau data on the medically uninsured simply can't be denied," Los Angeles Times, September 17, 2009; available at: http://articles.latimes.com/2009/sep/17/business/fi-hiltzik17

13 Michelle Fabio, "Is Your Child a U.S. Citizen if Born Abroad?" Legalzoom.com, October, 2007; available at: http://www.legalzoom.com/marriage-divorce-family-law/family-law-basics/is-your-child-us

14 John Lowell, "Consumer Driven Health Care-Who Are It's Users?" Employee Benefits Research Institute, May 27,2011; http://johnhlowell.blogspot.com/2011/05/consumer-driven-health-care-who-are-its.html

15 "IRS to Add 16500 agents to Enforce Health Insurance Mandate," The Liberty Journal, March 19, 2010; available at: http://thelibertyjournal.com/2010/03/19/irs-to-add-16500-agents-to-enforce-heath-insurance-mandate/

CHAPTER 6

1   Hinda Chaikind, Bernadette Fernandez, "Preexisting Exclusion Provisions for Children and Dependent Coverage under the Patient Protection and Affordable Care Act (PPACA)," Congressional Research Service, January 24, 2011; available at: http://www.primaryimmune.org/advocacy_center/pdfs/health_care_reform/PreExisting%20Exlusion%20Provisions%20for%20Children%20and%20Dependent%20Coverage%20under%20the%20Patient%20Protection%20and%20Affordable%20Care%20Act_20110207.pdf

2   Robert Longley, "About the United States Congress," About.com,; available at: http://usgovinfo.about.com/cs/uscongress/a/aboutcongress.htm

3   "What Triggers a Rescission of a Health Insurance Policy?" Attorney Pages; available at: http://attorneypages.com/hot/trigger-health-insurance-rescission.htm

4   Gregory Gambone, "What Is a COBRA Health Insurance Policy?" eHow; available at: http://www.ehow.com/about_6642077_cobra-health-insurance-policy_.html

5   Kathleen Parker, "Obama's Spin," Topeka Capital Journal, July 19, 2011; available at: http://cjonline.com/opinion/2011-07-18/kathleen-parker-obamas-spin

6   Michael Gomes, "PPACA's One Year Anniversary-In Retrospect," Benefits at Work, March 23, 2011; available at: http://tomdaly.wordpress.com/2011/03/23/ppaca%E2%80%99s-one-year-anniversary-in-retrospect/

CHAPTER 7

1   "The True Effects of Comprehensive Coverage: Examining State Health Insurance Mandates," Baton Rouge Area Chamber of Congress Issue Brief, May 21, 2009; available at: http://www.brac.org/uploads/IssueBriefStateHealthInsuranceMandatesFINAL.pdf

2   Thomas Capone, "Making Health Insurance More Accessible," The Foundry, May 13, 2011; available at: http://blog.heritage.org/2011/05/13/making-health-insurance-more-accessible/

3   Victoria Craig Bunce, JP Wieske, "Health Insurance Mandates in the States 2009," Council for Affordable Health Insurance, 2009; available at: http://www.cahi.org/cahi_contents/resources/pdf/HealthInsurance Mandates2009.pdf

4   "U.S. Breast Cancer statistics," BreastCancer.org, April 19, 20011; available at: http://www.breastcancer.org/symptoms/understand_bc/statistics.jsp

5   Allison Bell, "PPACA: Feds Add Contraception to Preventive Care package," Life and Health National underwriter, August 1, 2011; available at: http://www.lifeandhealthinsurancenews.com/News/2011/8/Pages/PPACA-Feds-Add-Contraception-to-Preventive-Care-Package.aspx

6   "The True Effects of Comprehensive Coverage: Examining State Health Insurance Mandates," Baton Rouge Area Chamber of Congress Issue Brief, May 21, 2009; available at: http://www.brac.org/uploads/IssueBriefStateHealthInsuranceMandatesFINAL.pdf

7   "U. S. National Debt 2010," The Economic Collapse, 2010; available at: http://theeconomiccollapseblog.com/archives/u-s-national-debt-2010

CHAPTER 8

1   Angie Drobnic Holan, "Health reform bill creates a health insurance exchange," PolitiFact, July 16th, 2009; available at: http://www.politifact.com/truth-o-meter/promises/obameter/promise/52/create-a-national-health-insurance-exchange/

2   Phil Galewitz, "Consumers Guide to Health Reform," Kaiser Health News, April 13, 2010; available at: http://www.kaiserhealthnews.org/Stories/2010/March/22/consumers-guide-health-reform.aspx

3   "Federal Employees Health Benefits Program Handbook," US Office of Personnel Management; available at: http://www.opm.gov/insure/health/reference/handbook/fehb02.asp

4 "A Detailed Timeline of the Healthcare Debate portrayed in 'The System'," Online Forum, 1994; available at: http://www.pbs.org/newshour/forum/may96/background/health_debate_page1.html

5 King Solomon, Ecclesiastes 1:9, NIV Bible; available at: http://www.biblegateway.com/passage/?search=Ecclesiastes+1%3A9&version=NIV

6 Robert Moffit, "Obamacare and Federal Health Exchanges: Undermining State Flexibility," The Heritage Foundation, January 18, 2011; available at: http://www.heritage.org/research/reports/2011/01/obamacare-and-federal-health-exchanges-undermining-state-flexibility

7 Robert Moffit, "Obamacare and Federal Health Exchanges: Undermining State Flexibility," The Heritage Foundation, January 18, 2011; available at: http://www.heritage.org/research/reports/2011/01/obamacare-and-federal-health-exchanges-undermining-state-flexibility

8 John Lowell, "Consumer Driven Health Care-Who Are It's Users?" Employee Benefits Research Institute, May 27,2011; http://johnhlowell.blogspot.com/2011/05/consumer-driven-health-care-who-are-its.html

9 Peter Grier, Health care reform bill 101: What's a health 'exchange'?" The Christian Science Monitor, March 10, 2010; available at: http://www.csmonitor.com/USA/Politics/2010/0320/Health-care-reform-bill-101-What-s-a-health-exchange

10 "American Cancer Society recommendations for early breast cancer detection," American Cancer Society, September 17, 2010; available at: http://www.cancer.org/Cancer/BreastCancer/DetailedGuide/breast-cancer-detection

CHAPTER 9

1 Suzanne Sataline, Shirley S. Wang, "Medical Schools Can't Keep Up," The wall Street Journal Health, April 12, 2010; available at: http://online.wsj.com/article/SB10001424052702304506904575180331528424238.html

2 "Solutions to the Challenges facing primary care medicine," American College of Physicians, 2009; available at: http://www.acponline.org/advocacy/where_we_stand/policy/solutions.pdf

3 American Association of Medical Colleges (AAMC), "Treating the healthcare crisis by increasing medical school enrollment," The Internet Medical Journal, 2008; available at: http://medjournal.com/wp/treating-healthcare-crisis-increasing/

4 "National Hospital Ambulatory Medical Care Survey: 2007 Outpatient Department Summary," National Health Statistics Reports, September 23, 2010; available at: http://www.cdc.gov/nchs/data/nhsr/nhsr028.pdf

5 "Advancing Primary Care," Council on Graduate medical Education-Twentieth Report, December 2010; available at: http://www.hrsa.gov/advisorycommittees/bhpradvisory/cogme/Reports/twentiethreport.pdf

6 Leigh Page, "New Medicare Physician Fee Schedule Includes 10% Increase for Primary Care, General Surgeons in Shortage Areas," Becker's Hospital review, November 15, 2010; available at: http://www.beckershospitalreview.com/hospital-financial-and-business-news/new-medicare-physician-fee-schedule-includes-10-increase-for-primary-care-general-surgeons-in-shortage-areas.html

7 Suzanne Sataline, Shirley S. Wang, "Medical Schools Can't Keep Up," The wall Street Journal Health, April 12, 2010; available at: http://online.wsj.com/article/SB10001424052702304506904575180331528424238.html

8 Katherine Mangan, "Medical-School Applications Barely Rise Even as Doctor Shortage Looms," The Chronicle of Higher Education, October 20, 2009; available at: http://chronicle.com/article/Medical-School-Applications/48880/

9 Suzanne Sataline, Shirley S. Wang, "Medical Schools Can't Keep Up," The wall Street Journal Health, April 12, 2010; available at: http://online.wsj.com/article/SB10001424052702304506904575180331528424238.html

10 Bradley Wertheim, "Congress must lift the cap on residency funding," Los Angeles Times/BuffaloNews.com, February 6, 2011; available at: http://www.buffalonews.com/editorial-page/viewpoints/article333368.ece

11 Alan Portner, "Doctor shortage may be mitigated by Nurse Practitioners and Physician Assistants," Examiner.com Wahshington DC, August 26, 2009; available at: http://www.examiner.com/public-policy-in-washington-dc/doctor-shortage-may-be-mitigated-by-nurse-practitioners-and-physician-assistants

12 Family Physician and Nurse Practitioner Training, "Nurse Practitioner Information Kit," American Academy of Family Physicians, available at: http://www.aafp.org/online/etc/medialib/aafp_org/documents/press/nurse-practicioners/np-training.Par.0001.File.tmp/NP_Info_FP-NP Training-Compare-4pgs.pdf

13 Gautham Nagesh, "Arizona doctor says Obamacare will force him to close shop," The Daily Caller, April 14,2010; available at: http://dailycaller.com/2010/04/14/arizona-doctor-says-obamacare-will-force-him-to-close-shop/

14 Peick Law Group, P.S. A Pacific Northwest Law Firm, Health Insurance Law, January 1, 2011; available at: http://www.peickconniff.com/

15 "Time Guideline for 99211, 99212, 99213, 99214, 99215 – E and M code," Medicare Fee Schedule, Payment and Reimbursement Benefit Guideline, CPT Code Billing, October 25, 2010; available at: http://www.medicarepaymentandreimbursement.com/2010/10/time-guideline-for-99211-99212-99213.html

16 Dr. Pullen, "How Can We Encourage Medical Students to Choose Primary Care? A Radical Suggestion – Pay Specialists Less," DrPullen.com, June 14, 2010; available at: http://drpullen.com/how-can-we-encourage-medical-students-to-choose-primary-care

17 Janice Lloyd, "Doctor shortage looms as primary care loses its pull," USA Today, August 18, 2009; available at: http://www.usatoday.com/news/health/2009-08-17-doctor-gp-shortage_N.htm

18 Sally C. Pipes, "The Doctor is Out-permanently," CA Political News, April 24, 2010; available at: http://capoliticalnews.com/blog_post/show/4938

19 Terry Jones, "45% of Doctors Would Consider Quitting if Congress Passes Health Care Overhaul," Investor's Business Daily, September 15, 2009; available at: http://www.investors.com/NewsAndAnalysis/ArticlePrint.aspx?id=506199

20 Sally C. Pipes, "The Doctor is Out-permanently," CA Political News, April 24, 2010; available at: http://capoliticalnews.com/blog_post/show/4938

21 Robert Lowes, "Stimulus Package Could Convert More Physicians to EHR's," Medscape Medical News Medscape Today, April 1, 2009; available at: http://www.medscape.com/viewarticle/590460

22 ScriptPad, " ScriptPad transforms your iphone and ipad into a digital prescription pad," 2010; available at: http://scriptpad.net/

23 Patient-Centered outcomes Research Institute (PCORI) Governing Board, September 23, 2010; available at: http://www.gao.gov/about/hcac/patientcentered_outcomes.html

24 Facts for Consumers, "Medical identity Theft," Federal Trade Commission, January, 2010; available at: http://www.ftc.gov/bcp/edu/pubs/consumer/idtheft/idt10.shtm

25 "Lifelock Receives Top Ten Ranking on Inc. Magazine's Inc 500 List," Identitytheftprotection.org, August 24th, 2010; available at: http://www.identitytheftprotection.org/identity-theft-protection-companies/lifelock.html

CHAPTER 10

1 "U.S. health care system: Worst in the world?" Washington Post, Seattle Post-Intelligencer, NPR; June 24, 2010; available at: http://theweek.com/article/index/204391/us-health-care-system-worst-in-the-world

2 Jessica Marshall, "U.S. Life Expectancy Lags in Most Counties," Discovery News, June 15, 2011; available at: http://news.discovery.com/human/us-life-expectancy-counties-110615.html

3   Robert Langley, "U.S. Infant Mortality Ranking Falls Again," About.com U.S. Government Info., October 21, 2008; available at: http://usgovinfo.about.com/b/2008/10/21/us-infant-mortality-ranking-falls-again.htm

4   The World Health Report, "World Health Organization assesses the World's Health Systems," The World Health Organization (WHO), 2000 Report: available at: http://www.who.int/whr/2000/media_centre/press_release/en/

5   Greg Soltis, "Consumable Camera to Offer Intestinal Tour," Live Science, June 19, 2008; available at: http://www.livescience.com/2631-consumable-camera-offer-intestinal-tour.html

6   "Murder Rate in the United States and Germany," Atlantic Review, October 5, 2006; available at: http://atlanticreview.org/archives/434-Murder-Rate-in-the-United-States-and-Germany.html

7   List of countries by life expectancy, 2005-2006, available: http://en.wikipedia.org/wiki/List_of_countries_by_life_expectancy

8   List of countries by infant mortality, 2011, available: http://en.wikipedia.org/wiki/List_of_countries_by_infant_mortality_rate

9   Krissi Danielsson, "Premature Birth and Viability," About.com Miscarriage/Pregnancy loss, August 15, 2008; available at: http://miscarriage.about.com/od/pregnancyafterloss/a/prematurebirth.htm

10 "Calgary's quads: Born in the U.S.A.'" The Calgary Herald, August 17, 2007; available at: http://www.canada.com/calgaryherald/story.html?id=41ccae74-8325-449a-b89f-e68957ca25ae&k=79546

11 "Infant Mortality and Premature Birth," BigGovHealth, Still Birth Definition Act 1992; available at: http://biggovhealth.org/resource/myths-facts/infant-mortality-and-premature-birth/

12 "Reducing Infant Mortality," CIA World Factbook, July 1, 2009; available at: http://nursingbirth.com/2009/07/01/coming-soon-free-movie-reducing-infant-mortality/

13 "Income, Poverty and Health Insurance Coverage in the United States: 2009," U.S. Census Bureau, September 16, 2010; available at: http://www.census.gov/newsroom/releases/archives/income_wealth/cb10-144.html

14 NHE Fact Sheet, Center for Medicare and Medicaid Services, 2009; available at: https://www.cms.gov/NationalHealthExpendData/25_NHE_Fact_Sheet.asp

15 1943:The Current Tax Payment Act, "Historical Perspectives on the Federal Income Tax," TaxHistory.com; available at: http://www.taxhistory.com/1943.html

16 "2010 Social Security Wage Base and FICA Tax Rate," American Payroll Association, October 15, 2009; available at: http://www.payrollexperts.com/BlogRetrieve.aspx?BlogID=3486&PostID=92248

17 Kate Pickert, "The Unsustainable U.S. Health Care System," Time Mobile, February 4, 2010; available at: http://swampland.time.com/2010/02/04/the-unsustainable-u-s-health-care-system/

18 CPR Statistics, CPR and Sudden Cardiac Arrest Fact Sheet, American Heart Association, April 26, 2010; available at: http://americanheart.org/HEARTORG/CPRAndECC/WhatisCPR/CPRFactsandStatistics_UCM_307542_Article.jsp

19 Kathleen Doheny, "Cancer Survival Rates Vary by Country," WebMD Health News, July 16, 2008; available at: http://www.webmd.com/cancer/news/20080716/cancer-survival-rates-vary-by-country

CHAPTER 11

1 "1968 New and Expanded Secretarial Powers Under the Health Reform Law," Health Reform Report, July 20, 2011; available at: http://healthreformreport.com/2011/01/1968-new-and-expanded-secretarial-powers-under-the-health-reform-law.php

2 "Neat Things About Paying for the Healthcare Bill-Facts and Convictions," Citizen 68, July 20, 2011; available at: http://www.citizen68.com/2010/03neat-things-about-paying-for-healthcare.html

3 "IRS Expansion," FactCheck.org, February 22, 2011; available at: http://www.factcheck.org/2010/03/irs-expansion/

4 Tory Newmyer, "Washington's most powerful women," CNN Money, 2010; available at: http://money.cnn.com/galleries/2010/news/1009/gallery.powerful_women_washington_dc.fortune/index.html

5   "CHT Reveals 1968 New and Expanded Secretarial Powers in Health Law, Center for health Transformation, 2011; available at: http://www.healthtransformation.net/cs/news/news_detail?pressrelease.id=3867

6   Cheryl Handy, "What is the Medicare Appeal Process?" eHow; http://www.ehow.com/how-does_5477080_medicare-appeal-process.html

7   "H.R. 3590; Sec. 3310. Reducing Wasteful Dispensing of Outpatient Prescription Drugs in Long-term Care Facilities Under Prescription Drug Plans and MA-PD Plans," NCPA LTC, August 27, 2011; available at: http://www.ncpaltc.org/index.php/short-cycle-fill/13-hr-3590-sec-3310-reducing-wasteful-dispensing-of-outpatient-prescription-drugs-in-long-term-care-facilities-under-prescription-drug-plans-and-mapd-plans

8   Newt Gingrich, "1968 Reasons to Repeal," Newt Gingrich Letter, January 19, 2011; available at: http://www.humanevents.com/article.php?id=41265

9   "Kansas Congressman Tim Huelskamp Calls on Secretary Sebelius to Let the Sun Shine on Waiver Process," Tim Huelskamp Website, June 6, 2011; available at: http://huelskamp.house.gov/index.php?option=com_content&view=article&id=3368

CHAPTER 12

1   Health Care, Carmen Group Incorporated; available at: http://www.carmengroup.com/healthcare/current-environment

2   "Obamacare," Intellectual Takeout; available at: http://intellectualtakeout.org/library/chart-graph/total-spending-under-ppaca-through-10-years-implementation?library_node=70586

3   Scott A. Hodge, "Tax Burden of Top 1% Now Exceeds That of Bottom 95%," Tax Foundation, July 29, 2009; available at: http://www.taxfoundation.org/blog/show/24944.html

4   "Requiring property ownership to vote," HubPages; available at: http://troylaplante.hubpages.com/hub/Requiring-property-ownership-to-vote

5 Jeanne Sahadi, "Medicare tax hikes: What the rich will pay," CNN Money, March 25, 2010; available at: http://money.cnn.com/2010/03/22/news/economy/medicare_tax_increase/index.htm

6 Solomon M. Mussey Office of the actuary, Centers for Medicare and Medicaid Services, April 22,2010; available at: https://www.cms.gov/ActuarialStudies/downloads/PPACA_Medicare_2010-04-22.pdf

7 "Summary of the patient Protection and affordable Care Act," Ortho World, 2010; available at: https://www.orthoworld.com/site/docs/op/online/2010/mayjun/editorial_ppaca.pdf

8 Blake Ellis, "Health care bill imposes 10% tax on tanning salon customers," CNN Money, March 24, 2010; available at: https://www.orthoworld.com/site/docs/op/online/2010/mayjun/editorial_ppaca.pdf

9 FDA Law Update, "New Taxes for Pharmaceutical and Medical Device manufacturers/Importers/Distributors," FDA Regulation Lawyer and Attorney, July 12, 2011; available at: http://www.fdalaw-blog.com/2010/04/articles/legislation/new-taxes-for-pharmaceutical-and-medical-device-manufacturersimportersdistributors

10 The Phrase Finder; available at: http://www.phrases.org.uk/meanings/the-pen-is-mightier-than-the-sword.html

11 "Obama talks about pacemakers," YouTube-Broadcast Yourself, July 20, 2011; available at: http://www.youtube.com/watch?v=NvM5uOasqCc

12 Brian Blasé, Rea Hederman, Jr., Paul Winfree, "The Uncertainty of Health Care Projections," The Heritage Foundation, September 23, 2010; available at: http://www.heritage.org/research/reports/2010/09/the-uncertainty-of-health-care-projections

13 "Big Changes to IRS Form 1099 in 2011, 2012," Investing Blog, May 2nd, 2010; available at: http://www.investingblog.org/archives/637/big-changes-to-irs-form-1099-in-2011-2012/

14 Grover Norquist, "Obamacare Packs Crushing new Taxes," Newsmax.com, January 14, 2011; available at: http://www.newsmax.com/GroverNorquist/obamacare-taxes/2011/01/14/id/382849

15 Ronald Bachman, "Healthcare Consumerism: The Future of Employment Based health Insurance Post PPACA," Health Transformation; available at: http://www.healthtransformation.net/cs/ ConsumerismCorner070910

CHAPTER 13

1 Gerard F. Anderson, "Hospitals Charge Uninsured and 'Self-Pay' Patients More than Double What Insured Patients Pay," Johns Hopkins Bloomberg School of Public Health, May 8, 2007; available at: http://www.jhsph.edu/publichealthnews/press_releases/2007/ anderson_hospital_charges.html

2 Medicare Claims Processing Manuel, Chapter 4 – Part B Hospital; available at: https://www.cms.gov/manuals/downloads/clm104c04.pdf

3 Douglas Perednia, "Overhauling America's Healthcare machine, an excerpt," Medpagetoday's KevinMd.com, 2011; available at: http:// www.kevinmd.com/blog/2011/04/overhauling-americas-healthcare- machine-excerpt.html

4 "Health Maintenance Organization Act of 1973," Wikipedia; available at: http://en.wikipedia.org/wiki/Health_Maintenance_Organization _Act_of_1973

5 Blue Cross and Blue Shield of Minnesota, May 31, 2011

CHAPTER 14

1 Lori Montgomery, "Proposed long-term insurance program raises questions," Washington Post Politics, October 27, 2009; available at: http:// www.washingtonpost.com/wp-dyn/content/article/2009/10/27/ AR2009102701417.html

2 "What is Long-Term Care?" Medicare.gov, The Official U.S. Government Site for Medicare; available at: http://www.medicare. gov/longtermcare/static/home.asp

3   Ron Lieber, "The Changes to Save a Big idea," The New York Times, April 29, 2011; available at: http://www.nytimes.com/2011/04/30/your-money/health-insurance/30money.html?pagewanted=all

4   Douglas Elmdorf, Report to Congress, Congressional Budget Office, November 18, 2009; available at: http://www.cbo.gov/ftpdocs/107xx/doc10731/Reid_letter_11_18_09.pdf

5   Akiv Roy, "Sebelius: CLASS Act Is "Totally Unsustainable," Mandate Possible," Forbes, February 23, 2011, available at: http://www.forbes.com/sites/aroy/2011/02/23/sebelius-class-act-is-totally-unsustainable-mandate-possible/

6   Sally Pipes, "America Needs A Great Deal Less ClLASS," Forbes, April 4, 2011; available at: http://www.forbes.com/2011/04/04/health-care-class-act-opinions-sally-pipes_2.html

7   "Boustany Pushes for Repeal of CLASS Act in ObamaCare," Press Release Distribution, April 15, 2011; available at: http://www.prlog.org/11440027-boustany-pushes-for-repeal-of-class-act-in-obamacare.html

8   Melanie Evans, "Forging the Way," Modern Healthcare, pp 6-7,18-24, August 29,2011.

CHAPTER 15

1   Douglas Elmendorf, "CBO's Analysis of the Major Health Care Legislation Enacted in March 2010," Statement from Congressional Budget Office, March 30, 2010; available at: http://www.cbo.gov/ftpdocs/121xx/doc12119/03-30-HealthCareLegislation.pdf

2   Phil Gingrey, Tim Murphy, "Repeal IPAB," GOP Doctors Caucus, June 17, 2011; available at: http://doctorscaucus.gingrey.house.gov/News/DocumentSingle.aspx?DocumentID=247696

3   Robert Lowes, "Will healthcare Reform Increase Medicaid Pay as Well as Enrollment," Medscape Today, March 23, 2010, available at: http://www.medscape.com/viewarticle/718673

4   "Congressional Update," Adams and Reese, LLP, January 26, 2011; available at: http://www.adamsandreese.com/congressional-update -01-26-2011/

5   Rachel Weiner, "Palin: Obama's 'Death Panel" Could Kill My Down Syndrome Baby," Huff Post Politics, August 7, 2009; available at: http://www.huffingtonpost.com/2009/08/07/palin-obamas-death-panel_n_254399.html

6   Ellen Meara, Meredith Rosenthal, Anna Sinaiko, "Comparing The Effects Of Health Insurance Reform Proposals: Employer Mandates, Medicaid Expansions, And Tax Credits," Harvard University, February 2007; available at: http://epionline.org/studies/meara_06-2007.pdf

CHAPTER 16

1   "It's the law of the land: Health overhaul signed," MSNBC, March 23, 2010; available at: http://www.msnbc.msn.com/id/35999823/ns/politics-health_care_reform/t/its-law-land-health-overhaul-signed/

2   Kyle Trygstad, "NBC/WSJ Poll: Only 33% Think Health Reform Is Good Idea," Real Clear Politics, January 19, 2010; available at: http://realclearpolitics.blogs.time.com/2010/01/19/nbcwsj-poll-33-want-health-reform/

3   Sean Duffy, "Most Americans Still Oppose PPACA," duffy.amplify, March 23, 2011; available at: http://duffy.amplify.com/2011/03/23/most-americans-still-oppose-ppaca/

4   Mark Ryan, "Rep. Ryan's Budget Plan Increases Support for the PPACA," National Physician's Alliance, June 12, 2011; available at: http://npalliance.org/blog/2011/06/12/rep-ryans-budget-plan-increases-support-for-the-ppaca/

5   Ronald Reagan, The Quotation Page; available at: http://www.quotationspage.com/quote/33742.html

6   Maggie Mahar, "A Reply to the CATO Institute," The Health Care Blog, July 16, 2010; available at: http://thehealthcareblog.com/blog/2010/07/16/a-reply-to-the-cato-institute/

7   Josie Raymond, "Government Health Spending to Surpass private Health Spending in 2012," News.change.org, February 5, 2010; available at: http://news.change.org/stories/government-health-spending-to-surpass-private-health-spending-in-2012

8   Barack Obama, "Barack Obama promises you can keep your health insurance, but there's no guarantee," PolitiFactCheck.com, August 11, 2009; available at: http://www.politifact.com/truth-o-meter/statements/2009/aug/11/barack-obama/barack-obama-promises-you-can-keep-your-health-ins/

9   "What does defensive medicine cost? It depends on your agenda," The Business Word, February 28, 2010; available at: http://www.business-word.com/index.php/weblog/comments/3378

10 "Want to cut costs in the ER? Pass medical liability reform," Texans for Lawsuit Reform, may 23, 2011; available at: http://www.tortre-form.com/news/want-cut-costs-er-pass-medical-liability-reform

11 "Surviving on a resident's salary?" ValueMD, April 4, 2006; available at: http://www.valuemd.com/residency-match-forum/109554-surviv-ing-residents-salary.html

12 Dave Ramsey, "Dave Ramsey's Envelope System," Daveramsey.com, September 5, 2009; available at: http://www.daveramsey.com/article/dave-ramseys-envelope-system/lifeandmoney_budgeting/

13 Thomas J. Stanley, "The Millionaire next Door: The Surprising Secrets of American's Wealthy," The New York Times on the Web; available at: http://www.nytimes.com/books/first/s/stanley-millionaire.html

14 Resource Center, "Health Savings Accounts," U.S. Department of the Treasury; available at: http://www.treasury.gov/resource-center/faqs/Taxes/Pages/Health-Savings-Accounts.aspx

15 "Health Savings Account Enrollment Reaches Ten Million," America's Health Insurance Plans, May 19, 2010; available at: http://www.ahip.org/content/pressrelease.aspx?docid=30516

16 "Changes are coming to a health care account near you," Wealth Informatics, September 22, 2010; available at: http://www.wealthin-formatics.com/2010/09/22/fsa-hsa-changes-2011-guidelines/

17 Robert Langley, "Congress Getting a Pay Raise-How About You?" About.com, January 3, 2009; available at: http://usgovinfo.about.com/b/2009/01/03/congress-getting-a-pay-raise-how-about-you.htm

18 The Declaration of Independence, "Life, Liberty, and the Pursuit of Happiness," Ayn Rand Center for Individual Rights; available at: http://principlesofafreesociety.com/life-liberty-pursuit-of-happiness/